Mysteries of Nutrition

An Easy Reference Handbook
For Those Who Nurture

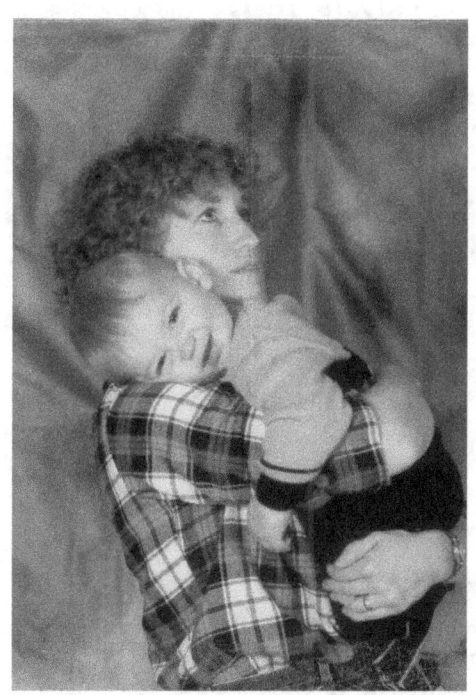

By Pop McCommon

2nd edition

Books by Pop McCommon:

<u>Personal Family Books Series</u>

Ancient Family Text – some history of the
McCommon/Nesmith families and an
autobiography of Pop McCommon

Ancient Family Journals – the journal stories of
two Nesmith sisters and other family data

Ancient Family Photos – the old family photographs
with captions and stories that describe them

For My Grandchildren – all the things Pop would
have said to his grandchildren but, because of
life circumstances, was unable to

The Will To Serve – Two extraordinary stories of
family members who lived ordinary lives

<u>Casual Discussion Series</u>

Keep Talking – contains the first six Casual
Discussion Books:

> **The Dark and the Light of the Moon**
> **Aged To Perfection**
> **The Teaching Art**
> **Natural Rhythms**
> **Being the Best You Can Be**
> **Challenges of the Ego**
>
> **Vanishing Point**

<u>General Topics</u>

East Side Poetry	**Flights of Fancy**
Tale of Two Women	**Solitude and Humor**
Mysteries of Nutrition	**Pop's Corner**

To my special friend, Fanny, who introduced me to good nutrition and healthy eating and who has, over the years, continued to monitor my good habits. From her I learned many things, two of which are to make ginger tea and to use turmeric in my cooking.

Introduction

As you go through life, you are educated about foods in various ways: school, T.V. shows, advertisements, newspaper and magazine articles, your family, friends, interest groups, and research studies. You hear many claims. Information that is good today is not good twenty years later. Sorting through information becomes tedious and most people don't bother.

Where it concerns the food we put into our bodies every day, it is hard to know what is true and what is false. Most of us want to treat ourselves well and stay healthy, yet there sometimes isn't enough good information that allows us to do that. For instance, we don't know what effects herbicides, pesticides, and fungicides have on the physical body when they spray them on our food supply. One popular chemical product is potent, extremely toxic, and can be taken up into the plant through the root system so that you can't wash it off. It is ingested with your food.

Much of what we hear has fear attached to it so that those who care often develop neuroses where eating is concerned. Treating eating disorders is a thriving business. I always wished I had a basic handbook that wasn't written in medical jargon or that didn't sound like propaganda. I didn't need the history of vitamins or the ways calcium is transported through cell walls.

My needs had to do with staying healthy and feeding people at my table, so I wished for a simple reference that could answer basic questions and keep me pointed in the right direction. Well, this is the book. I had to write one myself and it is well-researched.

Table of Contents

Mysteries of Nutrition

An Easy Reference Handbook
For Those Who Nurture

Chapter 1 Gaining An Understanding

Information about nutrition as found in this book is in the form of a general discussion since the subject of nutrition is always evolving with new discoveries and information. A general discussion tries to cover what is known at the present time, constituting our best knowledge to date, we hope. Experts in the field must remain open-minded for that reason. No one possesses a definitive answer, and there is no one formula that includes all people.

In any general discussion there are specific examples that do not apply. For instance, the nutrition of wheat grains does not apply to those with celiac disease, nor does the nutrition in dairy products apply to those with lactose intolerance. It is important to do your own thinking when reading any information so that what you apply from it makes good sense for you.

There are always those whose experience is outside the norm, so in a casual discussion which I hope this book represents even though much of the data is from professional books, we are talking about what we assume to be the majority experience based upon our best knowledge so far. If you are a small child, or pregnant, or elderly, if you have a genetic disorder or a chronic illness, then you have a special circumstance and it would be wise to educate yourself in order to determine the changes in diet that affect you.

We are supposed to be living in the present moment and making each present moment the best it can be at our present level of understanding. There are advantages to living in the present moment. Each present moment shows us that we are yet alive, that we have choices, that for most Americans we have food, clothes, shelter, companionship, and the natural environment with its rain, its flowers, and its sunshine. If we made each present moment the best it could be, life would seem so much more abundant. Part of utilizing the NOW moment is to pay attention to what fuel we feed our bodies so that in any present moment our minds are clear, our emotions are appropriate, and our energy level serves us.

One goal in writing this book was to get to the point quicker. As I read all that was written on food (until I'd had enough), I was frustrated continually with rhetoric that went on and on without seeming to arrive at the one piece of information I was looking for. A lot of every book seems to be filler, something to take up space so it can be called a book, and I feel not enough importance is given to the factual material. An author might explain to you that every word is factual and valuable, but factual or not, much of what is written is unnecessary unless you are a professional who specializes in a field the information applies to. The average guy or gal reading about food which is an everyday reality on the table is being taught about food by specialists and is left to decipher what is essentially a foreign language.

If the goal is to teach basics, or to reach the average American, the writing on the subject of food needs to be limited to what is important in human health, a good reference. With marketing propaganda, special interest manipulations, scientific compartmentalizing, the average person is kept confused or in the dark about what is really important and, instead, is given reasons to fear what "*may be important.*"

They use that term a lot: "may." It *may* be essential, it *may* lead to cancer, it *may* cause serious illness, it *may* have adverse consequences. You have to ask yourself how afraid would you like to be? The world "*may*" end tomorrow. It also *may not*. And, it *may not* cause cancer. A sure-fire way to get cancer is to become a worrier, afraid of living.

To top it off, you are referred to your doctor for further nutrition advice, which is funny, because doctors don't receive training in nutrition. If you take note of the number of doctors who drink and smoke and who are overweight, you might wonder if they are the best source for the information you need?

What usually happens is that without reliable information to go on, people fall back on what is familiar when eating foods, back to the training they received at home from parents. Home is where they felt safe, so what comes from the home has to be good, right? Moms, aunts, and grandmas have tried-and-true recipes they use. There are recipes for each holiday where pleasant things are associated with food. There are favorite recipes ("the best chocolate chip recipe ever!"), there are recipes that have been in the family "for generations." When you're a kid and your grandma makes donuts for you, you don't forget that! You remember that Mom's spaghetti is your favorite. Aunt Gertie made the *best* pie!

There are comfort foods, too. Mashed potatoes and gravy, perhaps, or Aunt Mazie's fried chicken. After every ball game our local softball team played, my dad made a pot of chili and we downed it with ice cold A & W root beer. You could count on a warm, sliced and buttered loaf of Grandma's banana bread to go with you when you went on the train. My uncle treated us with a freshly-caught plate of fried razor clams for breakfast whenever we visited.

The trick is to analyze the food you like to eat to see if it meets your requirements for good nutrition. If it does, great! If it doesn't, find out what could be added to make it nutritionally sound. That's why this book gives you the latest on vitamins and minerals, and why it talks about balance. You are then able to figure a lot out for yourself so that you are in charge of your own health where food is concerned.

People want to eat what they are used to, so it's hard to get them to like foods that they are unfamiliar with. The problem with what our parents taught us, or with comfort foods, they are often associated with bad habits that lead to disease states. Too much gravy for fifty years clogging arteries, for instance. However, consider that my grandparents lived into their eighties eating comfort foods and without the information in this book.

People will eat a known white bread and feel uncomfortable while eating Indian curry. The curried food is much better health-wise, but it's "different," so these people stick with what is known, even if it's not so good for their health. Your body adjusts and eliminates unused food to a degree.

One of the things that drives a bad habit is that you can't see the effects for a long time. It's like being young, you can't see how reckless behavior will affect you until it's too late. The young feel invincible, and that is how people feel about what their mothers said about food. Mom can't be wrong. Mom wouldn't hurt me.

Well, maybe not intentionally. Moms do their best with what they know and that's all you can ask of them, but knowledge is an evolving thing. If we received an education, we should be able to read what the latest is and, since we all have dealt with liars all our lives, we should be able to interpret what the media says about food.

It doesn't matter what the AMA or the USDA or any of the other corporate marketing divisions say with their food pyramids and charts and graphs. You can read nutrition books, like this one, and you can be in a program that eats "healthy," like weight watchers, or you can follow a diabetic menu. There are still oddities that crop up, reports of someone who did things differently, or results that didn't fit the norm.

An example, victims of the holocaust reported wearing thin pajama-type clothing and going barefoot in sub-zero weather while working under extreme conditions. Food for them was generally an unsavory soup and they said they "used to fight for the pea that floated on top." Add to those conditions the severity of the stress they were under with physical abuse and with all they had lost, including loved ones. When the survivors were finally released from captivity and were given a physical, many of them were found fit and in good health in spite of the conditions. In fact, many were more fit than the people who were not imprisoned!

How would one explain the health of people who were deprived? You wouldn't hear of a modern doctor prescribing deprivation as a program for good health, yet the experience of these survivors seems to suggest that there is more to physical health than food.

Another example, Inuit and Yupik Eskimos at one time were considered the healthiest people on the planet. They had little disease. Get this... their diet was 80% fat, seal oil, blubber (muk tuk), and so forth. Try that diet with our current no-fat, low-fat attitudes.

White men came along and changed the eating habits of the Eskimo to white man's food. Suddenly, they developed diseases and dental caries, things they hadn't had before. In order to cure them of cancer, doctors told them to go back to eating their traditional diet, and...it cured them. The cancers went away.

Australian Aborigines, as I understand it, don't have gardens, or supermarkets, or nutrition centers, or lobbyists in congress haggling over the label of "organic." They welcome the day with thanks for what they will receive, then as they walk about, any animal, snake, lizard, insect that crosses their path on that day can be used for food. It is gratefully accepted. There is a feeling that the animal crosses their path on purpose to be sacrificed as food, and that eating that animal is a positive act of exchanging energy.

Science tells us that energy can neither be created nor destroyed, it only changes form. Eating is changing the energy of the animal into the energy of the human. It is considered a sacred exchange. How would Americans fare with that diet?

Western cowboys existed on a fairly steady diet of beef and beans. How long do you think you could go with that diet? Slaves in the South were denied standard food, so ate the weeds, like peanuts, and the leftovers, like sow belly and chicken wings. Sailors are famous for contracting physical ailments when their diet does not include citrus. Prisoners of war eating only rice contracted beriberi. There are so many examples of eating habits and what happens physically as a result.

It is easy to see, as these types of examples come into our awareness, that there is more to food and eating than we have been taught. Of course, there are physical differences that can account for different diets and different disease states, different reactions to certain foods. Warm climates and cold climates require unique diets. Different cultures and races eat differently. The rich eat food that the poor can only dream of. There are actually genetic differences, even within families, that have one person eating a clam dinner while a sibling is deathly allergic to shellfish.

Research studies are sometimes very informative. Two that I can think of provide some new information I want you to have.

About ten years ago, I ran across a research study involving 40,000 participants of various groupings where they were looking to see which group was the least healthy, then drawing conclusions as to why it was so. I am not citing studies here as I assume my target audience would like to cut to the chase. This is an informal handbook so I'll just tell you what I read. Those so inclined can look elsewhere for particulars of studies.

Included in the study were groups like hikers, backpackers, vegetarians, vegans, probably raw food enthusiasts, barbequers, boaters, office workers, and so forth. Lots of groups. The results of the study surprised everyone! The study took in years of research and found that the least healthy group was 10 times more toxic than the second-rated group. The least healthy group was the backpacker-vegetarian group.

The backpacker-vegetarian group was assumed from the beginning to be the healthiest of all, yet the findings were the opposite. It was determined through further research that the reason that group scored so poorly was because they ate fruits and vegetables that had been regularly sprayed with pesticides and herbicides. Their bodies were storing the toxic chemicals. Not only that, toxins are stored in the fat of the body, and these people were habitually in the low-fat categories. In that case, toxins are stored in muscle and vital organs.

The other study I found interesting was for aluminum and how it acts around food. I grew up with many families owning aluminum cookware because it was so much lighter than cast iron, and it was common to wrap baked potatoes in aluminum foil, along with other leftovers.

What they did in the study was to pick up apples that had fallen from a tree, they tested them for the presence of aluminum, which initially was not present, and then they put them in an aluminum pot and set it under the tree on the ground for a period of several hours. They also tested the apples still in the tree. They were negative for aluminum.

After a period of time, the researchers came back and tested the apples again for the presence of aluminum and found the apples in the pot to be full of aluminum molecules. Not only that, they randomly tested the apples in the tree and found those apples to also be saturated with aluminum molecules.

The conclusion of the study was that aluminum should never be around food as it seems to be able to transfer molecules through the air. The presence of aluminum in food was suspected in the dramatic rise in the last fifty years of Alzheimer's and dementia. Aluminum attaches to brain cells. It is one of our minerals in food, as well as being a metal, but when aluminum is used around food we get an overdose, which has consequences.

As far as cookware goes, the use of cast iron will add iron to the food which is good for those with a tendency toward anemia. Stainless steel has not shown any adverse effects for food that I am aware of, but it's worth staying tuned to new information to find out if that holds true.

What you should know about cooking is that heat causes your pan and the food in it to exchange atoms. Much of the exchange is also with the water in the pan, so that when you throw out cooking water, you are throwing out many nutrients. It would be good if you could reuse the water for other dishes, or in baking. I make soups out of it.

Another tip, when you buy canned fruit, buy the kind packed in it's own juice, without added sugar, then use the juice as water in Jello. Using Jello to add fruit to is one way to get your children or husband to eat fruit that they wouldn't otherwise want to eat. Add roasted pecans, berries, and sunflower seeds, too. The sugar in Jello is undesirable but you pick your battles. If it gets people eating more fruit...? It doesn't fit with a no-sugar diet, but it does fit with a plan of moderation in all things.

When you eat raw vegetables, you get more of the vitamins. When you cook them, you get more of the minerals. You win either way.

High heat kills especially the water-soluble vitamins, vitamin C and vitamin B complex. From best to worst ways to cook from what I have read: baking, stir-frying (low temp.), boiling, broiling, barbequing, frying, deep-frying, microwaving. Raw will always be best but it must be balanced with some cooked food. Key word: balance.

There is another element to eating that isn't usually thought of but is very important. There are studies that show human emotions can transfer to food. There are well-documented studies of the effect of human thought on water crystals, with surprising results. There are actual chemical changes altering the food. You would have to believe that the Aborigines knew what they were doing when they welcomed any "food" that crossed their path during the day, and that the Native Americans knew what they were about when they said a prayer for the animal after a kill.

So, while your food is being prepared, you might want to ensure harmony in your house. A fight with your wife and then not talking during dinner is going to put food in your system that can be toxic, or at the very least, not usable for your body. Emotions can nullify the effects of nutrients. One father I knew regularly grumbled about how terrible his wife's cooking was and, one time, threw the food he didn't want against the wall, shattering her grandmother's china. Do you think, in that case, food is being digested well?

One way for couples to set a good example for their children is to happily prepare food together, one blending a recipe while the other dices vegetables. Soon, you will have kids helping and when the family participates in an activity together, you already know that's a healthy situation.

If you are a thinking person, information is always changing, so it is important to keep up with it. That's why we learn to read in school and communicate, our education is expected to help keep us informed. Read food labels. It is our responsibility to inform ourselves since we are responsible for the welfare of our children. It becomes a skill to interpret the information on a food label.

The vitamin and mineral part of the book is organized like so:

A page or two for each vitamin and each mineral. This includes information on what the particular element does for the body, why we need it, what happens if we don't get it (then, for fun, try to explain to yourself the health of Natives who had a diet of 80% fat) and any other pertinent information that might be helpful.

Once you learn where the nutrients are in food, you can make a shopping list of the things you are willing to eat. Vegetarians will leave out meat, but then must decide what will replace meat as a protein food, like a combination of beans and rice, or corn and rice. Vegans will leave out anything artificial, or with animal sources. Gluten-intolerant people will leave out most grains. Lactose-intolerant people will leave out dairy. Those with hyperactive children will leave out sugar.

Diabetics will expand the taboo on sugar to other sweeteners and fruit, as well.

If you want *a good core food group* to work with, no matter who you are, try to become very good at fixing **vegetables**. They will never steer you wrong unless they are not organic. Then chemical toxins are a problem. Add to vegetables **seeds** and **nuts** and **herbs**, always looking for organic types. Use **coconut oil** for cooking, or light **olive oil** which handles higher temperatures better. Use dark olive oil as a salad dressing.

With the vegetable group, add in whatever else makes you feel healthy according to your individual philosophy of eating. You want beer or wine? You want donuts? You want thick steaks? The rule is *"everthing in moderation."*

Couple your **diet** with a good core lifestyle, plenty of **rest** and **exercise**, along with whatever gives you **peace of mind**, and it won't matter which road you take with eating, you will find health. All diets are different steps on the road to awareness and growth. We learn at our own levels, with our own body types, then grow more as we become more knowledgeable. Your human body will make adjustments as you develop health awareness. Everyone is different and we do not have to all believe the same way. We are individuals, always.

I kind of wanted a handy reference for this information that didn't take hours of my time to wade through. Even when I found a good book on the subject, it was written for professionals or it contained a lot of stuff I didn't need to read. Now I have this book. You're welcome!

Chapter 2 Available Information

Who do you listen to when it comes to nutrition ? Interest groups abound!

One of your choices is *corporate America* which regularly puts out information designed to promote their profit margins. They really aren't interested in nutrition or good health, or in you. They deal in marketing products.

Another of your choices is the *medical establishment*. They profit from illness, so they regularly play down the benefits of good nutrition as a factor in promoting good health. They give lip service, yes, but too little follow-through. Doctors aren't trained in nutrition yet they are whom you are sent to for advice. Nurses get nutrition training, but their training is watered down under the withering stare of the medical model. Also, the AMA does not honor research that is done by those outside of their purview, no matter how prestigious the work.

A third choice is *the FDA* which sets standards for vitamin/mineral consumption. They have the annoying habit of treating everyone as if they are the same, that the needs of a 300 lb. sumo wrestler are just slightly higher than the needs of a ninety-pound elderly woman. Few distinctions are made so that every teen is the same, every pregnant woman is the same, every senior citizen is the same. They are also subject to the influences of lobbyists for both corporate America and the medical establishment.

Choice number four, you can take a class in or attend a workshop or conference on nutrition. Who it is that teaches it and where the college, workshop leader, or lecturer gets its funding will determine how accurate the information is. You can either become very informed with vital information attending these workshops, if you are fortunate, or you can get the usual status quo information, the watered down kind.

You can also have **choice number five**, self-educating. If you know how to research, you can learn a lot this way. There is a lot of good information currently in print.

If you don't know how to research, here are a few clues.

*1 Use as many sources as possible – to write this book I used between fifty and sixty sources of information representing different nutritional philosophies. I used over a hundred research studies.

Most people go to church, so let me put it to you in those terms: if you want to know the probable meaning of any Bible verse, first read it in context, then use a dozen different translations. If you can find gospels that weren't included by the councils of Nicaea, and if you can peruse the Dead Sea Scrolls and other ancient documents, you'll be even closer to finding meaning. Hopefully, you get the picture. It takes a lot of **good information** coupled with an **open mind**.

*2 There is so much written, volumes upon volumes, on the subject of nutrition that you should severely limit your search to the most important things you want to know, otherwise you will be deluged with more than you can handle and easily overwhelmed to the point of exhaustion. Unless you live in a monastery away from all distractions and research is your job, you won't have the time.

*3 Pay attention to who is doing the talking in the literature. If they belong to or support special interests, the information won't be accurate. Also, there are researchers who have limited their research parameters as I have advised you to do, and while they can talk with authority about the material they covered, they are usually not in possession of all the facts. That applies to everybody, including me. You have to have an attitude of leaving your mind open for more information as it becomes available. This book represents the best I can give you at this point in time. Twenty years from now, or tomorrow, much of it could change. If you use what is here as a guide, it will keep you alive and well even if, later, some of the details change.

I would like to add a note here, an important one. Our environment is so polluted that we can't trust our food, our water supply, the air we breathe, and there are even chemicals in our clothing and other things that touch our skin. We are inundated by radiations from technology and EMF's from cell towers, etc. You get the picture. The average person has two choices:

1) be afraid of everything and slowly give up hope because of how overwhelming the problem is, or be angry about it and do nothing, letting the anger make you unhealthy, or

2) learn how to survive it. The place you start is with something we do every day, eat and drink. That's what this book addresses.

Vitamins

Chapter 3 Vitamins

There are two basic types of vitamins: water-soluble and fat-soluble. It has to do with storage. Water-soluble vitamins leave the body through the urine and sweat if there is more than enough. Fat-soluble vitamins, when there is plenty, are stored in the body to be used when needed.

Because fat-soluble vitamins, A, D, E, K, are stored, it would be easy to get too much of these vitamins, like when eating a bunch of carrots turns your skin orange, so you don't necessarily need to eat them every day. Water-soluble vitamins, C and B complex, are usually not toxic in quantity, although it is still possible to get too much, just not generally done.

Vitamins that come in food take care of themselves. They work together, have a check and balance system, and it's real hard to overdose on any of them when they're in food.

Vitamin supplements should be taken with plenty of water as B and C are diuretics, that is, they ask the body to lose water. If you don't get enough water with vitamin supplements, or by the way, with coffee or colas, you run the risk of kidney stones and other ailments. Vitamins ideally should come from your food.

B vitamins and vitamin C are excreted by the body when in excess, in the feces, urine, perspiration, and tears, and can be variously harmed by light, high temperatures, and cooking with water. They team with enzymes to do much of the energy work in the body.

The following information is presented in brief form in order to expedite the finding of pertinent information. Recommended FDA daily amounts are listed first with the subtitle.

Recommended amounts are for the average man or woman for sedentary activity, but amounts vary slightly for body size, vigorous exercise, the elderly, children, teens, alcohol & drug use, and pregnant or lactating women.

Basic List of Vitamins

<u>Water Soluble Vitamins</u>:

B1 – thiamin
B2 – riboflavin
B3 - Niacin
B5 - Pantothenic Acid
B7 - Biotin
B6 – pyridoxine
B9 - Folate – folic acid
B12 – cobalamin
C – ascorbic acid

As was stated, water soluble vitamins leave the body daily through sweat, feces, urine, tears, therefore they need to be replaced.

Vitamin C is considered a master vitamin and is needed for others to work properly. B vitamins are essential for normal metabolism, red blood cell formation, and immune and nervous system functioning.

Metabolism is the physical and chemical burning of energy to achieve transformations.

<u>Fat Soluble Vitamins</u>:
A, D, E, K

Fat-soluble vitamins are stored in body tissues like muscles and the liver until needed, therefore the need for them is not the same as for water-soluble vitamins.

Vitamin A - Fat Soluble – 5,000 IU/day

Uses of vitamin A
*essential for growth; *good vision; *maintenance of skin cells; *maintenance of soft tissue membranes; *health of gums and teeth; *resistance to bacterial and viral infections; *health of glands; *protein synthesis; *effects of smoking; *effects of aging; *health of reproductive organs; *prevention of birth defects; *handling stress.

Deficiencies of vitamin A
*stunted growth; *vision problems and blindness; *skin diseases; *dental abnormalities; *problems with sex glands, uterus, bladder, urinary tract; *bone pain; *abnormal fetus, or fetal death; *predisposition to tuberculosis; predisposition to cancer; disease states.

Toxic situations that deplete vitamin A
*poor eating habits; *smoking; *nitrates and nitrites; *air pollution; very high protein intake; *extreme temperatures.

Common Foods with vitamin A
Plant sources: carrots; squash; pumpkin; apricots; peaches; yellow corn; sweet potatoes; melons; broccoli; dried prunes; green leafy vegetables; asparagus; tomato juice.

Animal products: meat; cod liver oil, milk, cheeses; eggs; butter.

You are trying to balance vitamin A that comes from plants and vitamin A that comes from animal products for good health. Some of each is desirable. If you are vegetarian or vegan, a good knowledge of nutrition is needed to compensate. The human body does not produce adequate vitamin A from precursors like carotene from plants alone.

Expanded Notes for vitamin A

*What isn't circulated in the bloodstream to be used by cells is stored in the liver.

*Very high doses are toxic.

*Nitrates are found in fertilizers mostly of commercially-grown plant crops. When they are stored, they form very dangerous nitrites. The longer the storage, the more nitrites. Nitrites destroy vitamin A in both the blood stream and in storage. Usually found in tap water and processed meats, but can be in any food, even baby foods.

*Air pollution uses up vitamin A which tries to support tissues and membranes to resist pollution. Hard on respiratory system.

*Viruses can't reproduce on their own and must enter the body's cells and take over the cell reproductive processes. Vitamin A strengthens cell walls so that viruses and bacteria can't penetrate.

*Important to thymus gland which can produce more antibodies against disease. Important to thyroid and adrenal glands which speed oxidation of food in winter to preserve body heat.

*Vitamin A is important for protein synthesis and both are required for growth. A high protein diet needs to have increased amounts of vitamin A. They work together.

*Vegetarians/vegans need more vitamin A to synthesize plant proteins. (important)

*Aging symptoms like vision, hearing, and smell loss may be corrected with vitamin A.

*deficiencies have been associated with tired and aching eyes after close work, burning and itching eyes, sensitivity to light, reduced vision or irreversible blindness, spontaneous abortion, failure to conceive, impotence, birth defects, absence of limbs, heart anomalies, and cleft palate.

Side Note

*We said earlier that the diet of the healthiest people in the world was composed of 80% fat. That might make you curious, as it did me. Think about that fats are needed for vitamin A to work. Vitamin A also works hand-in-hand with protein. Fats are the group that is needed to survive in survival situations, which is why Green Berets and others are taught to eat insects and grub worms, as they are nearly 100% fat. In extreme cold, extra vitamin A is needed, so an Eskimo diet is good for Eskimos. Fish provide the other nutrients.

* Vitamin A breaks down or turns rancid with light and higher temperature, so most vitamin A foods are found in the refrigerator. Basically, foods containing vitamin A actually contain vitamin A components, like carotene, that are then converted to vitamin A in the intestinal wall and liver of the body, or when animals eat plants, a conversion takes place in their bodies. That's how meat can have vitamin A.

*Think of vitamin A foods as being orange, red, and dark green as a general rule.

Vitamin B1 – Thiamine – Water Soluble
1.5 mg to 2.3 mg/day

Uses of vitamin B1 (Thiamin)

*promotes appetite; *provides better digestion; *promotes growth; *fights the effects of alcohol; *essential in carbohydrate metabolism; *used to transmit nerve impulses; *needed for oxidation of cells.

Deficiencies of vitamin B1

*Overall numbness and tingling; *cramping pain in legs; *difficulty walking; *severe heart problems; *extensive tissue damage; *fatigue; *lowering of stamina; *irritability; *depression; *liver disease; *weight loss; *paralysis; *beriberi; *death.

Toxic Situations

None

Common Foods with vitamin B1

Plant sources - *whole grains, especially oatmeal; *potatoes; *beans; *peas; *nuts; *peanuts; *cold cereal; *seeds; *crackers; *orange juice; *wheat germ; *brewer's yeast; *green, leafy vegetables

Animal products - *organ meats; processed meats, like hot dogs; *pork (a huge B1 source); *dairy products; *eggs.

Expanded Notes on vitamin B1

*discovered while looking for a cure for beriberi

*beriberi is severe disabling outcome involving paralysis and death

*higher temperatures and soda will kill B1

*loss of vitamin by 1/3 when boiling; in meats, loss of 60% when roasting, 30% when broiling, 15% when frying, and bread baking 5-15% loss. This will be true of all other water-soluble vitamins with varying percentages when cooking. There will be losses.

*at most risk when deficient are alcoholics, drug addicts, those living in poverty.

*canned food will suffer loss of water-soluble vitamins when packed in liquid

*severe problems happen when processed grain, rice are used as staples of diet.

*You need more thiamin if

- there is excess sugar and starch in your diet

- you are cooking with water

- if you are in your golden years

- you are pregnant or lactating

- you have a fever

- you just had surgery

- you are under stress

- you have greatly increased physical activity

Side Notes

* B vitamins treat a variety of nerve and mental disorders

* B1 helps with myasthenia gravis and early multiple sclerosis

Vitamin B2 – Riboflavin – Water Soluble
1.5-2.0 mg/day

Uses of Vitamin B2 (riboflavin)
Vitamin B2 promotes: *growth; *reproductive health; *stamina; *oxidation process in tissues; *metabolism of fats, carbohydrates, and amino acids in protein.

Deficiencies of Vitamin B2
*stunted growth; *abnormal skeleton; *low stamina; *increasing weakness; *digestive disturbances; *moody, nervous, tired; *hair loss; *sore mouth and nose; *eye burning, inflammation, vision dimness, conjunctivitis, cataracts; *anemia (happens with low B2, folic acid, and iron); *dermatitis, scaly skin patches around mouth, genitals; serious impairment of liver; *personality disturbances; *birth defects; *paralysis; *death.

Toxic Situations
None

Common Foods with vitamin B2
Plant sources: *yeast; *whole grains; *green leafy vegetables; *sprouting seeds; *beans; *peas; *nuts; *fruits; *wheat germ.
Animal sources: *liver; *organ meats; *other meats; *dairy products, especially milk; *egg yolks; *cheese.

Expanded Notes
*"flavus" in riboflavin means "yellow," so...riboflavin...flavanoids...refers to color of pigment in the vitamin
*people most at risk for deficiencies are alcoholics and athletes who don't drink milk

*a high meat diet can offset low dairy intake; this is quite often the case with athletes

*most deficiency symptoms can be reversed with treatment of correct vitamins

*excess B2 is stored in muscle tissue

*can be destroyed by light, alkaline solution, antibiotics, alcohol, oral contraceptives, so those on contraceptives, along with vegan diets need to use fortified sources to meet needs.

Side Note

*All information that applies to human nutrition also, in general, applies to animals, like your pets. Exceptions have to do mainly with nutrients animals can produce in their body that humans can't. *Pet nutrition* is important, so careful study of what applies to your pet is recommended.

*"Synthesis" is a word that is used a lot in nutrition. It has to do with the formation of a complex compound by combining two or more simpler compounds. In other words, using parts to make a whole.

Niacin – Water Soluble – 20 mg/day

Uses of Niacin

Niacin promotes: *cellular metabolism; *carbohydrate/fat/protein synthesis; *health and growth of tissues; *appetite and proper functioning of digestive tract; *utilization of food in the body; *normal functioning of the brain.

Deficiencies of Niacin

Deficiencies cause: *widespread changes in the body; *dermatitis, especially where skin is exposed to the sun; *poor appetite; *weight loss; *weakness; *diarrhea, abdominal pains, and other gastrointestinal disturbances; *sleeplessness; *rashes; *nervous tissue problems; *mental disturbances, like dementia; *pellagra (means rough or painful skin); *death.

Toxic Situations

none; slight burning or itching sensations in doses over 100 mg/day

Common foods with niacin

Protein sources in general are good sources.

Plant sources: *asparagus; *mushrooms; *peanuts; peas; *sunflower seeds; *whole wheat flour; *Brewer's yeast; *whole grains; *green leafy vegetables.

Animal sources: meat, fish, organ meats; milk; *eggs.

Expanded Notes

*Heat stable, so little is lost in cooking unless cooking water is thrown out. Ideally, cooking water should be reused for soup stock

or in mixing ingredients to retain use of the nutrients

*Niacin lost with use of oral antibiotics

*Doses over 100 mg/day are sometimes given medically to lower cholesterol levels as it helps blood vessel dilation

*Most deficiencies happen where there were poor standards of living and where corn was a staple of the diet.

*Those at risk for deficiencies: alcoholics; those with refined diets where niacin is destroyed by processing

Side Note

*An increase in carbohydrates robs niacin.

*Daily requirements for a person has a lot to do with how much muscle mass there is in each individual. More muscle, more of a need.

*Deficiencies can be mistaken for mental illness, like a lot of B vitamins, which is why mental institutions are fewer now. They gave B vitamins to the insane and discovered that many were cured enough to go home.

*Can be used to treat schizophrenia.

Vitamin B6 – (Pyridoxine) - Water Soluble –
2 mg/day

Uses of vitamin B6
Vitamin B6 promotes: *formation of adrenaline and insulin hormones; *carbohydrate/fat/protein metabolism; *most important in iron and potassium metabolism; *synthesis of neurotransmitters, hemoglobin, white blood cells, RNA, and DNA; *needed for production of antibodies and red blood cells; *helps with tooth decay.

Beneficial for asthma, rheumatism, kidney stones, atherosclerosis, cancer immunity, PMS, menses, and acne.

Deficiencies of vitamin B6
Deficiencies cause: *widespread symptoms, like impaired immune response, skin disorders, mental confusion and depression, and anemia; *vomiting; *nerve irritation; *headaches; *seizures; tics, tremors, twitches.

Most prevalent deficiency in the U.S. Deficiencies found in Down's Syndrome, mongolism, rheumatoid arthritis, diabetes, and aging.

Toxic Situations
2-6 g/day for a prolonged period can potentially cause walking difficulties and irreversible nerve damage.

Common Foods with vitamin B6
Plant Sources: most fruits and vegetables, especially like bananas, cantaloupe, broccoli, spinach, soybeans, walnuts, peanuts, peas,

brown rice, sunflower seeds, Brewer's yeast, wheat germ.

Animal Sources: beef, fish, poultry.

Expanded Notes

*most at risk: alcoholics, those on cortisone, and pregnant women

*heat, cooking, processing, storage destroy vitamin B6

*stored in muscles

*B6 from animal sources is absorbed better than from plants

*B6 is a catalyst that makes many things work

*a high protein diet takes the B6 from other areas leaving a deficiency in those areas

*for cramps and spasms, use B6 with calcium, magnesium, and potassium.

*often taken as a supplement during difficult menses

Side Note

*B6 activates many enzymes. Enzymes, for those who are unaware, are responsible for carrying out the activities of living cells. Our bodies are composed of cells. Enzymes stimulate chemical transformations from the nervous system, to the heart, to emotions. They continually evolve, like a set of tools that seek to improve themselves. Enzymes bind together all living things and processes, maintaining the unity of life at the molecular level.

Pantothenic Acid – Water Soluble - 10 mg/day

Uses of Pantothenic Acid

Pantothenic acid promotes: *release of energy from carbs/fats/proteins; *protection against allergic reactions and radiation damage; *tissue regeneration; *mitigation of toxic substances, like antibiotics; *relief of gas in the gut; *decrease in grinding of teeth at night.

Deficiencies of Pantothenic Acid

Deficiencies cause: *burning foot syndrome;" *numbness, tingling, shooting pains in the extremities; *arthritis, especially rheumatoid and osteo-types; *mental and neurological symptoms; *headache; *sleep disturbance; *nausea; *muscle cramps; *impaired motor coordination; *weakened resistance to stress and infections; *birth defects, stillbirths, mental retardation; *fatigue; *stomach distress; *constipation; *ulcers; *glandular disturbance.

Amazingly, with all they know about what deficiencies do, deficiencies are listed as rare!

Toxic Situations

None

Common Foods with Pantothenic Acid

Plant Sources: *mushrooms; *peanuts; *soy flour; *dark buckwheat; *sunflower and sesame seeds; *most vegetables; *nearly all fruits; *sweet potatoes; *broccoli; *Brewer's yeast; *wheat bran.

Animal Sources: *liver; *organ meats; *other meats; *lobster; *milk; *eggs; *mother's milk.

Expanded Notes on Pantothenic Acid

*Insecticides and other chemicals destroy pantothenic acid.

*Processing of foods, refining, freezing, canning, cooking, antibiotics can all cause losses, but pantothenic acid found in all foods of the four food groups.

*Alcoholics, the poor, and the elderly at risk for deficiencies.

Side Note

*You don't often run across a vitamin that can have a positive effect on a condition like the grinding or gnashing of teeth at night, called bruxism, but pantothenic acid, with calcium, is the real deal, according to the studies I read. It needs to combine with calcium, iodine, and vitamins A, C, and E, but the combination of those nutrients apparently takes care of or greatly reduces the problem.

*Life can be stressful so it is important to pay attention to how often you laugh, use humor, move around like in dancing, get enough sleep, reduce stress, and relax doing things that are fun. Quieting the mind is essential daily. Appreciate beauty and see it everywhere. Love yourself enough to show respect in the way you live. Good feelings digest food well and promote nutrition.

Biotin – Water Soluble – 300 mcg/ day
(mcg = microgram)

Uses For Biotin

Biotin promotes: *carbohydrate and fat metabolism; *synthesis of glucose, fatty acids, and DNA; *the breakdown of amino acids; *normal growth.

Deficiencies for Biotin

Deficiencies cause: *scaly inflammation of skin; *pathological changes in tongue and lips; *decreased appetite; *sleeplessness; *anemia; *nausea and vomiting; *depression; *muscle pain; *weakness; *poor growth.

Here again, like with pantothenic acid, many deficiencies are listed, yet a deficiency of biotin is considered unlikely. Enough requirements are apparently found in the diet.

Toxic Situations

Unknown, but it is known that raw egg consumption inhibits absorption of biotin, with a possible side effect of salmonella.

Common Foods with Biotin

Plant Sources: *cauliflower; *nuts; *brown rice; *rolled oats.

Animal Sources: *meats; *fish; *egg yolks; *cheese; *milk; mother's milk.

Expanded Notes for Biotin

*alcoholics are at risk for deficiency
*stable to heat
*deficiencies can be induced with cooking, antibiotics, and sulpha drugs.

Choline – Water Soluble – requirements unknown

Uses for Choline
Choline promotes: *every bodily function; *nervous system; *healthy liver; *immune response; *lifelong resistance to disease combined with folic acid, vitamin B12, and an amino acid; *resistance to cancer.

Deficiencies for Choline
Deficiencies cause: *weakness; *listless; *muscle and nerve damage; *accumulation of fat in the liver; *increased blood pressure, headache, dizziness, palpitations; *constipation; *gland abnormalities; *body diseased by poisons; *paralysis; *cardiac arrest; *death.

Toxic Situations Unknown

Common Foods with Choline
Plant Sources: *lecithin; *soybeans; *Brewer's yeast; *wheat germ; *peanuts.
Animal Sources: *fish; *liver; *egg yolk; *breast milk.

Expanded Notes for Choline
*they are still researching this vitamin
*needed for nerve impulses so nerve impulses can jump the synapse
*too many sugar/alcohol calories use up choline so it is not available to do jobs elsewhere.

Side Note
Breast milk is rich with most vitamins and minerals.

Folic Acid (Folacin) – Water Soluble –

180-200 mcg/day

Uses for Folic Acid

Folic acid promotes: *DNA and red blood cell formation; *cell division; *wound healing; *the mitigation of the effects of food poisoning, blood clots, heart attack, stroke; *healing of schizophrenia.

Deficiencies of Folic Acid

Deficiencies cause: *insufficient DNA resulting in anemia; *poor white blood cell formation; *inflammation of the tongue; *poor growth; *diarrhea; *problems with nerve function; *vomiting; *hair loss; *birth defects; *mental illness; *poor healing and resistance to infection; *toxemia; *premature birth; *heart palpitations; *headaches.

Toxic Situations None

Common Foods with Folic Acid

Plant Sources: *green leafy vegetables; *sprouts; *asparagus; *orange juice; *wheat bran; *turnips; *potatoes; *black-eyed peas; *lima beans; *chard; *broccoli.

Animal Sources: *organ meats, especially liver.

Expanded Notes for Folic Acid

*alcoholics and pregnant women, the poor, elderly, teens are at risk for deficiencies

*food preparation and processing destroys 50-90% of folic acid; should steam or stir fry; oral contraceptives, air, light, antibiotics, sulpha drugs, all destroy folic acid

*losses during pregnancy increase birth defects.

Vitamin B12 – Water Soluble – 6-15 mcg/day

Uses of Vitamin B12

Vitamin B12 promotes: *neural functions, maintaining the myelin sheath insulation around nerves; *folic acid metabolism; *blood health; *growth; *conversion of carbs to fats; *carbohydrate/fat/protein utilization; *resistance to germs; *fertility; *works as a master nutrient affecting many systems.

Deficiencies of Vitamin B12

Deficiencies cause: *weakness; *back pain; *chronic fatigue; *difficulties walking; *stammering; *jerking of limbs; *damage to nervous system, like with pernicious anemia which destroys the nerves; *reduced DNA/RNA; *permanent mental deterioration; *paralysis; *cerebral or spinal lesions; death.

Toxic Situations None

Common Foods with Vitamin B12

Plant Sources: Brewer's yeast.
Animal Sources: *liver; *clams; *oysters; *hot dogs; *beef; *pork; *eggs; *milk; *organ meats; *fish; *crab; *cheese.

Expanded Notes for Vitamin B12

*found in animal sources; there is no good plant source; vegetarians and vegans must use fortified cereals and breads
*alcoholics, those with liver disease, the elderly, pregnant women, those on the pill, children, the poor, vegetarians, and vegans are all at risk for deficiencies.
*binds with protein in saliva, released for absorption by stomach acid.

Vitamin C – (Ascorbic Acid) – Water Soluble –
60-500 mg/ day

Uses of Vitamin C

Vitamin C promotes: *synthesis of the protein, collagen; *connective tissue, bones, teeth, tendons, blood vessels; *healing of wounds; *iron absorption; *the fight against cancer; *prevention of colds and other infections; *detoxifying of toxic substances; *the reinforcement of the body's defenses; *moderation of cardiovascular disorders, infectious diseases, cancers, collagen diseases, the effects of aging, all forms of diabetes, carbon monoxide, damage caused by burns, gallstones, blood clot formation, immune system disruptions, scurvy, frostbite, fractures, eye cataracts, memory loss and abnormal brain activity, bleeding gums, diarrhea, and high cholesterol.

Deficiencies of Vitamin C

Deficiencies cause: *problems with all of the above.

Toxic Situations None

Common Foods with Vitamin C

Plant sources: most fruits and vegetables, but specifically, *citrus fruit; *green peppers; *cauliflower; *broccoli; *cabbage; *strawberries; *papayas; *romaine lettuce; *potatoes; *leafy green vegetables; *grapefruit; *tomatoes; *tangerines; *spinach; *kale; *blueberries; *cantaloupe; *Brussels sprouts; *avocados.

Animal Sources: none

Expanded Notes for Vitamin C
   *master vitamin; needed in the diet
   *easily lost in processing and cooking
   *smokers need more as vitamin C is pulled from other areas to fight the effects of smoking; also true for alcohol
   *others at risk for deficiency are the poor, the elderly, infants, diabetics, teens, those exposed to chemicals and drugs, those who use aspirin regularly like with arthritis, and pregnant women
   *treating burns with vitamin C has been in spray form and works well
   *bike riders who have to bike along roadways with car exhaust might want to consider increasing their dose of vitamin C
   *up to 140,000 mg/day has been given to fight severe pneumonia; normal cold/flu 2-3,000 mg/day, less for children

Side Note
   Linus Pauling and several other prestigious individuals have done extensive research on vitamin C using higher doses, up to 4,000 mg/day per individual and more, and they were unable to find any ill effects at higher dosages. They even used themselves as guinea pigs in the experiments. However, their work has not been honored by the establishment. There is a lot of infighting in the medical and scientific community over vitamin C, a lot of posturing and territorialism, as is normal for those groups. I tend to agree with Pauling (et al) since they are the ones who won Nobel Prizes for their research. I personally take 1000-2000 mg/day and went from yearly colds, flu, and bronchitis to *no* sickness for the last thirty years.

Para-aminobenzoic Acid (PABA) – Water Soluble
Requirements unknown

Uses for PABA
PABA promotes: *the stimulation of other vitamins; *the metabolism of protein; *the production of blood cells; *the prevention of skin cancer and other skin conditions; *factors in healthy growth.

Deficiencies of PABA
Deficiencies cause: *digestive disorders; *nervousness; *depression; *skin ailments.

Toxic Situations
Unknown

Common Foods with PABA
Plant Sources: *Brewer's yeast; *wheat germ; *molasses.
Animal Sources: *liver; *eggs.

Expanded Notes for PABA
*sulpha drugs will nullify PABA
*still researching other benefits/problems

Still researching. New vitamin.

Side Note
*Water is the source of life. We are about 70% water so the work of the cells and pH balance require us to keep a good water balance. Being tired and dry mouth are indicators that you may need water. Make sure your water supply is safe. When in doubt, boil it or filter it.

Bioflavanoids (also known as Vitamin P;
Vitamin C2) –Water Soluble – requirements unknown

Uses for Bioflavanoids
Bioflavanoids promote: *most things in combination with vitamin C; *the strength of the body's capillaries; *improvement of venous tone; *mitigation of the pain from varicose veins; *is a potent anti-thrombosis agent.

Deficiencies of Bioflavanoids
Deficiencies cause: *skin disorders; *diabetic retinitis; *bleeding gums; * hemorrhoids; *skin easily bruised; *heavy menstrual bleeding, nose bleed, postpartum bleeding, and spontaneous abortion.

Toxic Situations
None

Common Foods with Bioflavanoids
Plant Sources: same foods as vitamin C, most fruits and vegetables with the white pulp in citrus fruits and bell peppers, also in red onion, thyme, parsley, blueberries, black tea, wine, cocoa.
Animal Sources: none

Expanded Notes for Bioflavanoids
*found in nature paired with vitamin C
*has a symbiotic relationship with legumes
*helps prevent disease of plants
*is the part of plants that attracts pollinators
*still researching

Inositol – Water Soluble – requirement unknown

Uses for Inositol
Inositol promotes: *low cholesterol levels; *brain function; *control of abnormal fats; *inhibitory effect on cancer; *growth factor; *important protective functions; *treatment of nerve damage, cirrhosis, and psoriasis.

Deficiencies of Inositol
None reported, but you can guess that the benefits above would cease to be benefits.

Toxic Situations   None

Common Inositol Foods   Animal Sources

Expanded Notes for Inositol
*still researching complex relationships.

* vegans need not worry; the body produces enough

Side Note
We have mentioned the metabolism of carbohydrates, fats, proteins a lot and here's why. Those are the principle structural components of cells and they are, by far, the most abundant nutrients in food. *Metabolism* is the burning of carbohydrates with fats and proteins in your bodies for energy. Think of a wood stove or fireplace in your home where you burn fuel for energy in the form of heat. Think of protein as the hardwood log you place on the fire that burns all day. Think of complex carbohydrates, like potatoes, rice, whole grains, vegetables, and fruits, as that soft-wood log (alder, pine, fir) that burns half-a-day. Think of fats as that wadded-up newspaper and kindling you used to get the bigger logs to catch fire, and think of simple carbohydrates, like junk food, candy, and soda, like maybe tissues or paper that burst quickly into flame and flare up for a brief period before being totally consumed and dying out just as quickly. They are good for a burst of energy if it is brief.

Vitamin D – Fat Soluble – 1000 IU/day

Uses of Vitamin D (called the "sun" vitamin)

Vitamin D promotes: *prevention of cancer, arthritis, and MS; *calcium absorption; *bone mineral metabolism and bone formation and density; *development of certain cells.

Deficiencies of Vitamin D

Deficiencies cause: *rickets (in children); *osteomalacia (adult rickets); possibly hardening of the arteries and retardation.

Toxic Situations

*4 or 5 times the recommended amount causes over-absorption of calcium and calcium deposits in body organs, causing metabolic disturbances and cell death. Intake needs to be monitored over 1000 IU/day. Dietary sources can be quite toxic; it's better to get it from sunlight.

Common Foods with vitamin D

*fish oils; *fortified milk; egg yolks.

Expanded Notes for vitamin D

*exposure to sunlight produces vitamin D on the skin

*younger people and whites need less exposure (15 min./day), seniors and darker skinned people need more; those who live in cloudy, smoky, foggy, colder environments need more

*at risk are those who don't get much sun, those who live where air is polluted, and those with vague, generalized aches and pains with muscle weakness that feels like rheumatism

Vitamin E – 400-800 IU/day – Fat Soluble

Uses of Vitamin E

Vitamin E promotes: *boost of selenium efficiency; *relieves pain from menopause; *helps varicose veins; *helps vitamin A absorption; *helps in detoxifying the body; *helps skin abnormalities; helps aging process, keeps cells younger longer; *boosts energy levels; *protects cell membranes; *maintains oxygen levels where needed; *helps to avert miscarriage; *increases stamina; * decreases anemia; *helps prevent blood clots; restores capillary permeability* protection against air pollution; *regulates levels of coenzyme Q; *healing of burns; *warts disappear; *increased alertness and learning ability; *fights cancer and muscular dystrophy, and periodontal disease; *helps prevent and heal heart attack; *helps prevent diabetic artery narrowing; *increases blood supply.

Deficiencies of Vitamin E

Deficiencies cause: disturbances of metabolism; *problems leading to sterility, impotence, or habitual abortion; *anemia; *low birth weight; *cell membrane breakdown (hemolysis); *blood clots; *atherosclerosis; *muscular dystrophy; *fetal death.

Toxic Situations with Vitamin E

Only a possible headache, diarrhea, nausea above 800 IU has been recorded in some people with average use. Doesn't include medical emergency use. Use cautiously with elevated blood pressure and chronic rheumatic heart disease.

Common Foods with Vitamin E

Plant sources: *leafy greens of many plants; *whole grains; *vegetable oils; *fresh and frozen spinach, asparagus, broccoli, cabbage; *wheat germ oil; *rice; *oats; *peanuts.

Animal sources: none

Expanded Notes

* Those most at risk: premature babies; those with faulty fat absorption like with liver cirrhosis and post-gastrectomy; those with obstructive jaundice, pancreatic insufficiency, sprue, and calf pain while walking.
* Vitamin E easily destroyed in cooking processes and prolonged storage.
* The leaves of vegetables are where it is found more than in the vegetable.
* Vitamin E is an antioxidant.
* Works with selenium: more E, less selenium; more selenium, less E
* People with phlebitis generally take supplements.
* Benefits for memory, emotions, allergies, stress; omega 3's; Alzheimer help.

Side Note

*Controversies exist with vitamin E because nutritionists and nutrition science in general have a set philosophy that everyone should be the same, thus the FDA requirements. Their tendency is to say if you don't have this amount, you can be harmed, which is a scare tactic. We are all individual and have different requirements. The trick is to eat healthfully and listen to your body. It will tell you through bitter taste, numbness and tingling around the mouth, nausea, diarrhea, headache, blurred vision, low energy, allergic reactions, and a host of other symptoms if something is wrong with what you are ingesting. The experts are a guide to use, but not an ultimate authority. If they were, their requirements and information wouldn't keep changing every few years.

Even open-minded scientists are confused about the unusual behavior of vitamin E since it is dependent upon nutrient partners that behave in a complicated way. Nutrient partners are often selenium, vitamin C, and vitamin A. The efficient body systems are linked to these partnerships.

There is a strong correlation between vitamin E and heart disease. It is been adequately shown in many, many studies that when there is a deficiency of vitamin E, the incidence and probability of heart disease rises.

Vitamin E is considered in research as a "broad spectrum" nutrient in that it is used successfully to treat many, seemingly unrelated, medical conditions. You can see by the multiple uses above that it is important to good health. Fortunately, we generally can get enough vitamin E even though much of it is destroyed in cooking.

Antibiotics is, however, one of the things that puts everybody at risk for deficiencies in many vitamins. Vitamin E acts as a natural antibiotic. The right diet would preclude the use of medical antibiotics in a perfect world.

Vitamin K – 60-80 mcg./day – Fat Soluble

Uses of Vitamin K
 * the clotting of blood

Deficiencies of Vitamin K (unlikely)
 * uncontrolled bleeding

Toxic Situations none; diet provides enough

Foods with Vitamin K
 Plant sources: *fresh food, like leafy greens, peas, green beans, spinach, cabbage, carrots, tomatoes, cauliflower, potatoes, soy beans.
 Animal sources: *liver; *lean meats.

Side Note: don't take supplements as there is enough of this vitamin found in food, especially if you are on blood-thinning medications.

Minerals

Chapter 4 Minerals

Minerals perform so many important tasks that they can't be ignored even though with many of them we only need trace amounts. The absence of several important minerals will result in the death of the human body. There are many that affect pregnancy and lactation.

Minerals are divided up into two main categories: sort of a main, heavy-hitting group that multi-tasks, and trace minerals. *Trace minerals* are described as all those we use at the level of 100 mg/day or less. They are all vital to human health or they wouldn't be in this book.

There are some other minerals that may make the list in some future time They are aluminum (which can be toxic in higher doses), antimony, arsenic (believe it or not! "Please eat your arsenic, honey, it's good for your health!"), barium, beryllium, boron, bromine, cadmium, cesium, germanium, gold, lithium, rubidium, titanium, and vanadium. These were mostly considered to be pollutants in food, but further research is revealing that they may play key roles in the human body at trace amounts. Pretty soon, if this continues, we'll have the whole chemical periodic table that is represented in a nutritionally healthy food plan!

The thing with vitamins and minerals is that their roles in human health are constantly evolving. Much research continues so that, perhaps in 20 years, this book will be completely out-dated. For now, it is a boiled down version of what is available to the average person who is not working in a scientific or medical field.

Main nutrients where daily requirements are more than 100 mg/day are: calcium, magnesium, phosphorus, potassium and sodium. These are the multi-taskers.

Trace minerals where daily requirements are considered at or less than 100 mg/day are: chlorine, chromium, cobalt, copper, fluorine, iodine, iron, manganese, molybdenum, nickel, selenium, silicon, strontium, sulfur, tin, and zinc.

All minerals work as a team with one or more minerals and vitamins so that a deficiency begins a cascading effect toward a disease state. For some nutrients the pace is rapid, for others slowly over time, but all need course corrections as we plan our diets.

Minerals, as you will undoubtedly notice, can be gotten from food, and also from environmental sources, such as from burning fossil fuels, from water softeners, or from processing of food, even from the water out of your tap. Some nutrients from these sources are used by the body in a healthy way while others do harm, causing toxic levels. It's good to know the difference.

Calcium – Up to 1400 mg/day

Uses for Calcium

Calcium promotes: *healthy bones, collagen (connective tissue, cartilage), and teeth; *nerve impulse transmission, essential to nerve cells that power breath, brain, muscle; *pairs with exercise to build bone; *regulates growth of glands; *aids clotting of blood; *aids muscular contractions; *aids cell metabolism.

Deficiencies of Calcium

Deficiencies cause: *abnormal growth; *without vitamin D, osteoporosis; *periodontal disease; *without vitamin A, adult rickets; *aggravated MS; *aggravated muscle cramps; *aggravated arthritis.

Toxic Situations with Calcium

*kidney stones in susceptible people; *bone spurs; *poor mineral absorption.

Common Foods with Calcium

Plant sources: *dark green leafy vegetables; *potatoes; *root vegetables; *blackstrap molasses; *artichokes; *beans; *whole grains; *nuts; *seeds; *tofu.

Animal sources: *bones (boiled); *dairy (a most important source); *eggs; *sardines; *salmon.

Expanded Notes

*groups at risk are women in general and the elderly

*there are many individual differences with calcium need; water softeners leach calcium if you have one; much is lost in sweat, and from inactivity, emotional stress, sleep disturbance *what you are used to will affect your dosage level, so use judgment when deciding how much you need based on how often you experience broken bones, bone/ joint/muscle pain, cramping, inflammation of your gums

*women in general need more than average

*cooked dandelion greens are an excellent source of calcium, but spinach/Swiss chard, and beet greens are a poor source as they contain oxalic acid that inhibits calcium

*estrogen replacement therapy is used to retard bone loss in post-menopausal women; those not replacing estrogen should be consuming 1500-2500 mg/day of calcium; those with therapy should still have 1000 mg/day of calcium

*remember, ice cream (and others) may be a good source of calcium, but it also has salt, fat, sugar, and artificial ingredients; so don't be afraid to eat ice cream, just remember that everything is balance. Moderation is the key.

Magnesium – Men 350/women 280 mg/day

Uses for Magnesium
Calcium promotes: *nerve and heart function; *activation of enzymes; *bone strength; bronchial dilation, so helps asthma sufferers.

Deficiencies of Magnesium
Deficiencies cause: *weakness; *muscle pain; *poor heart and nerve function; *lower blood pressure; *seizures; *irregular heartbeat; *disorientation.

Toxic Situations with Magnesium
Only with those who have kidney disease.

Common Foods with Magnesium
Plant sources: *green vegetables; *whole grains; *nuts; *legumes; *seeds; *chocolate (from the chocolate plant).
Animal sources: *milk; *meats.

Expanded Notes
*derived mostly from plant sources; found in plant chlorophyll
*groups at risk include women and people on thiazide diuretics
*over 300 enzymes use magnesium
*a condition like convulsions can be caused by low magnesium, but also by low vitamin B6; they both need to be present because they work together
*water softeners rob water of magnesium and calcium, and add sodium in large quantities which raises blood pressure

Phosphorus – 1500 mg/day

Uses for Phosphorus
Phosphorus promotes: *bone and tooth strength; *cell and cell membrane function; *metabolism as it is part of a variety of metabolic compounds; *aids enzyme function.

Deficiencies of Phosphorus
Rare, possibly some elderly women

Toxic Situations with Phosphorus
None

Common Foods with Phosphorus
Plant sources: *bakery products
Animal sources: *dairy; *meats.

Expanded Notes
*at risk groups include premature infants, the elderly, alcoholics, those with nutrient-poor diets, those who use aluminum-containing antacids, those whose medications contain aluminum, and vegans

*phosphorus likes to pair with vitamin D to get work done

*enzymes break down protein from food, so then fats and carbohydrates combine with phosphorus

*phosphorus also combines with B vitamins for effective use of both

*in processed foods, phosphorus is out of control and inhibits calcium

Sodium – 500 mg/day

Uses for Sodium
Sodium promotes: *fluid balance; *nerve impulse transmission.

Deficiencies of Sodium
Deficiencies cause: *muscle cramps.

Toxic Situations for Sodium
Hypertension leading to other major health issues, like atherosclerosis, heart attack, and stroke.

Common Foods with Sodium
table salt and processed foods

Expanded Notes
*if you own a water softener, you may want to consider using it for all water except drinking water and set up a drinking system that will bypass the water softener, such as a water cooler or bottled water
*group at risk is the group that is severely trying to restrict salt from their diets to lower blood pressure; easy to get too much sodium in our society

Side Note
Consider that natural foods have enough sodium already. Salt is used in processing and preserving. Salt is added to water by many cooks to make it boil quicker. Salt is added while preparing the meal. Salt is added again at the table. Can you see why people have high blood pressure (hypertension)?

Potassium – 2000 mg/day

Uses for Potassium
Potassium promotes: * fluid balance; *nerve impulse transmission.

Deficiencies of Potassium
Deficiencies cause: *irregular heartbeat; *loss of appetite; *muscle cramps.

Toxic Situations with Potassium
None

Common foods with Potassium
Plant sources: *fruits; *spinach; *squash; *tomatoes; *potatoes; *other vegetables.
Animal sources: milk

Expanded Notes
*Sodium and potassium are called electrolytes because they carry a small electrical charge in water. This is important in cell function as the difference in electrical charges with potassium on the inside of the cell and sodium on the outside of the cell create the transportation system of nutrients through permeable cell walls
*groups at risk for deficiencies are those in poverty and alcoholics

Zinc – 10-30 mg/day – trace mineral

Uses for Zinc

Zinc promotes: *fat/carbohydrate/protein metabolism; *wound healing; *strong bones and eyes; *tissue repair; *night vision; *healthy prostate; *reduction in inflammation; *reduction in body odor and acne; *resistance to infection; *immunity boost; * over 200 enzymes need zinc.

Deficiencies of Zinc

Deficiencies cause: *skin rash; *diarrhea; *hair loss; *decreased appetite and ability to taste; *poor growth and development; *poor wound healing; *decrease in HDL and increase in cholesterol numbers.

Toxic Situations for Zinc

*decreased iron and copper absorption; *diarrhea; *depressed immune function

Common Foods with Zinc

Plant sources: leafy greens; *whole grains; *beans; *peanuts; *peas

Animal sources: *milk; *yogurt; *sea foods like oysters, shrimp, and crab; *beef and other meats

Expanded Notes

*best absorbed from animal sources

*groups at risk for deficiencies are vegetarians, women, the elderly, the poor, the growing child, dieters, alcoholics

*unleavened bread is high in phytic acid which inhibits zinc

*parasitic infections, eating clay, some antacids all contribute to a zinc deficiency

Copper – 2 mg/day – trace mineral

Uses for Copper
Copper promotes: *red blood cell synthesis; *energy (iron) metabolism; *aerobic performance in the body; *blood clotting; *immune system function; *calm nerves, clear thinking; *keeps coronary arteries strong.

Deficiencies of Copper
Deficiencies cause: *anemia; *poor growth; *decrease in white blood cell count.

Toxic Situations for Copper
*nerve disorders; *vomiting; *mental degeneration; *triggers genetic Wilson's Disease

Common Foods with Copper
Plant sources: *cocoa; *beans; *nuts; *whole grains; *dried fruits
Animal sources: *liver

Expanded Notes
*Wilson's Disease can be treated
*groups at risk for deficiencies are premature infants, those recovering from intestinal surgery, and people who are overzealous in using zinc supplements

Iron – 200-400 mg/day – trace mineral

Uses for Iron
Iron promotes: *oxygen transport/delivery during exercise; *increased endurance; *decreased fatigue; *immune system function

Deficiencies of Iron
Deficiencies cause: *anemia and other blood disorders

Toxic Situations for Iron
Toxic to kids and those with hemochromatosis, a genetic disorder

Common Foods with Iron
Plant sources: *spinach; *broccoli; *peas; *bran; *enriched breads
Animal sources: *seafood; *liver and other meats

Expanded Notes
*women need more than men
*groups at risk for deficiency are infants, preschool kids, adolescents, child-bearing women, vegans
*best from animal sources; vegans and vegetarians should take vitamin C to supplement plant sources
*phytic acid, found in the husks of grains, grain fiber, tannins found in tea, oxalic acid found in certain vegetables, and some antacids all interfere with iron, zinc, magnesium, calcium absorption, but a high fiber diet of many varied vegetables usually provides enough minerals to compensate; most documented deficiencies recorded in cultures with 80% diet of unleavened bread

Selenium – 70-100 mcg/ day – trace mineral

Uses for Selenium
Selenium promotes: *protection against exercise injury; *decrease in fatigue; *activation of RNA/DNA; *manufacture of antibodies; *cancer protection.

Deficiencies of Selenium
Deficiencies cause: *muscle pain; *muscle weakness; *heart disease.

Toxic Situations for Selenium
Nausea, vomiting, hair loss, weakness, liver disease

Common Foods with Selenium
Plant sources: *whole grains; *seeds
Animal sources: *organ meats; *eggs; *fish; *seafood

Expanded Notes
*at risk groups unknown
*high fat foods are low in selenium
*fish with whole grains increases selenium
*selenium is an antioxidant

Chromium – 50-200 mcg/day – trace mineral

Uses for Chromium

Chromium promotes: *carbohydrate metabolism; *an increase in the effects of insulin; *decreases fatigue; *control of blood glucose levels.

Deficiencies of Chromium

Deficiencies cause: *increase in blood glucose levels after eating; *increase of blood cholesterol; *convulsions in infants; *factors leading to both heart disease and diabetes.

Toxic Situations for Chromium

Toxicity usually due to industrial contamination, not diet, leading to liver damage and cancer

Common Foods with Chromium

Plant sources: *mushrooms; *whole grains; *brewer's yeast; *plant nutrients tied to soil quality

Animal sources: *egg yolks; *cheese; *liver, pork and other meats

Expanded Notes

*at risk groups include people eating totally prepared foods and the elderly with non-insulin dependent diabetes

Silicon – unknown RDA dose –trace mineral

Uses for Silicon

Silicon promotes: *lower cholesterol levels; *lower heart attack risk; *stronger connective, soft tissue, and blood vessels; *with calcium, growth in bones and collagen.

Deficiencies of Silicon

Deficiencies cause: *none noted.

Toxic Situations for Silicon

None

Common Foods with Silicon

Plant sources: *foods high in plant fiber; *prunes; *sweet potatoes; *apples; *cooked spinach; *potatoes; *almonds; *plums; *beans; *corn; *peas; * blackberries; *lentils; *fruit; *coconut; *cooked broccoli; *raisins; *zucchini; *carrots; *squash; *also, drinking water.

Animal sources: none

Expanded Notes

*no at risk groups except if diet is devoid of fiber

*high fiber diet, meaning high selenium, lowers heart attack risk and cholesterol, as well as colon cancer, leading killers in our society

Manganese – 2-5 mg/day – trace mineral

Uses for Manganese

Manganese promotes: *action of some enzymes, like in carbohydrate metabolism; *with vitamin K, blood clotting; *bone formation and formation of connective tissue; *neurotransmitters communication between brain and body.

Deficiencies of Manganese

Deficiencies cause: *none, but sometimes implicated in epilepsy, lack of coordination of muscles, and twitching.

Toxic Situations for Manganese

Can be toxic at high doses so caution is recommended with supplement use.

Common Foods with Manganese

Plant sources: *whole grains, like rice, oats, along with wheat germ and wheat bran; *nuts; *beans; *sweet potatoes; *leafy greens; *prunes; *peas; *fresh fruit
Animal sources: liver

Expanded Notes

*at risk groups unknown

Iodine – 150-400 mcg/day – trace mineral

Uses for Iodine
Iodine promotes: *hormone synthesis; *growth and metabolism.

Deficiencies of Iodine
Deficiencies cause: *goiter; *poor fetal growth in the womb; *fetal retardation.

Toxic Situations for Iodine
Can be toxic in amounts over 1 mg. as it inhibits thyroid function

Common Foods with Iodine
Plant sources: *iodized salt; *plants and water near oceans; *kelp (use kelp in moderation)
Animal sources: *saltwater fish; *dairy

Expanded Notes
*also providing iodine are drugs, food additives, rainfall inducing silver iodide, and the burning of fossil fuels
*no longer deficiencies in America due to iodized salt
*those pregnant or breastfeeding need 175-200 mcg/day, but take great care in the dose as a fetus has little tolerance for deficiency or overdose
*iodine is part of the thyroid hormone

Cobalt – 3 mcg/day – trace mineral

Uses for Cobalt
Cobalt promotes: *vitality to all body cells, especially red blood cells.

Deficiencies of Cobalt
Deficiencies cause: *pernicious anemia; *fatigue; *diarrhea; *heart palpitations; *numbness in fingers and toes.

Toxic Situations for Cobalt
Irreversible brain damage, poor growth and mental development

Common Foods with Cobalt
Plant sources: *tempeh
Animal sources: *beef; *liver; *lamb; *tuna; *chicken; *cheese; *yogurt; *eggs.

Expanded Notes
*vegetarian/vegan diets need supplementation with B Complex or Brewer's yeast
*those at risk are newborns, children, and vegetarian/vegans

Fluorine (fluoride) – 1.5-4 mg/day – trace min.

Uses for Fluorine
Fluoride promotes: *strong teeth and bones; *resistance to tooth decay.

Deficiencies of Fluorine
Deficiencies cause: *greater risk of dental cavities.

Toxic Situations for Fluorine
*greater than 6 mg/day causes staining and mottling of teeth during development; *stomach upset; *bone pain; *weak bones and adult rickets

Common Foods with Fluorine
Plant sources: *tea; *seaweed; *brown rice; *potatoes; *oatmeal; *apples; *cooked spinach and kale; *soybeans
Animal sources: *canned ocean fish; *eggs; *cod; *mackerel; *beef; *chicken; *whole milk; *liver

Expanded Notes
*fluorine also available from fluoridated water, toothpaste, and dental treatments
*children are group most at risk, but also those who live in areas where there is no fluoridation, and those who lack dental treatment
*if your children's teeth become stained or mottled, it is because of too much fluoride in your drinking water; reduce the fluoride exposure and the staining will correct itself

Chlorine (chloride) – 700mg/day – trace min.

Uses for Chlorine

Chlorine promotes: *digestion; *immunity and nerve function; *cell health; *stomach acid production; *health of cerebral and spinal fluid; *water balance.

Deficiencies of Chlorine

Deficiencies cause: *unknown

Toxic Situations for Chlorine

When combined with sodium in susceptible people increases blood pressure

Common Foods with Chlorine

Plant sources: *table salt; *some vegetables; *processing of bread and vegetables.

Animal sources: *animal sources are the richest.

Sulfur – no RDA amount – trace mineral

Uses of Sulfur
Sulfur promotes: *drug detox, called a toxin bouncer; *acid-base balance

Deficiencies of Sulfur
Deficiencies cause: *none

Toxic Situations for Sulfur
None

Common Foods with Sulfur
Plant sources: in this case, plant combinations *legumes and whole grains or nuts; *eggs or other protein foods with grains; *beans and corn; *beans and rice; *rice and chili; *peanut butter and whole grain bread; cereal and milk; macaroni and cheese
Animal sources: *meats

Expanded Notes
*sulfur is a key ingredient in vitamins and amino acids
*groups at risk are vegetarians and vegans unless they know to use food combinations

Molybdenum - .15-.5 mg/day – trace mineral

Uses for Molybdenum

Molybdenum promotes: *action of some enzymes; *interaction with iron and copper and mobilizes iron from the liver; *rids the body of toxic nitrogen wastes from protein digestion; *dental enamel.

Deficiencies of Molybdenum

Deficiencies cause: *none except when there is a strict intravenous diet

Toxic Situations Unknown

Common Foods with Molybdenum

Plant sources: *beans; *whole grains; *nuts; *green leafy vegetables
Animal sources: *meats

Strontium – 20 mg or less/day – trace min.

Uses for Strontium
Strontium promotes: *bone and teeth health; *actions like calcium with decrease in tooth decay and bone loss; *cell/energy health

Deficiencies of Strontium
Deficiencies cause: *none

Toxic Situations for Strontium none

Common Foods with Strontium
Plant and animal sources: a good balance of usable protein

Expanded Notes
*we have heard that strontium 90 is radioactive but it is a by-product of nuclear fission, man-made splitting of the atom; strontium in nature is not radioactive
*found only in combination

Other Trace Minerals we are still learning about:

Tin	**Cesium**
Nickel *3-17 mg/day*	**Germanium**
Boron	**Rubidium**
Arsenic	**Titanium**
Cadmium	**Tungsten**
Lithium	**Beryllium**
Barium	**Antimony**
Bromine	**Aluminum**
Gold	
Vanadium *100-300 mcg/day*	

Chapter 5 Label Reading

In America, we have agencies who are responsible for labels on food. They are the FDA (Food and Drug Administration), who are responsible for food labels, the USDA (Department of Agriculture), who regulate meat and poultry, and the Bureau of Alcohol, Tobacco, and Firearms which oversees alcoholic beverages. In addition, the FTC (Federal Trade Commission) regulates the advertising of food products.

It used to be that listed ingredients in food were simple and in English, such as milk, eggs, sugar, salt. The order of ingredients listed on a label tells you what is the largest amount, in this case, milk. Salt would be the least amount in this example.

Then, ingredient lists had to have a breakdown of sugars and salts, as well as preservatives and additives, like guar gum, malt sugar, sodium benzoate, and whole milk solids. As manufacturers learned how to market to get around regulations, they began listing ingredients by their scientific designations, such as with malto-dextrin, disodium-phosphate, Red 40, Yellow 6, BHA, adipic acid, corn syrup powders, and hydrogenated vegetable oils.

The whole idea is to confuse the consumer so that they can't figure out what they're buying. The smiling housewife and wholesome scenery that usually advertises the item, plus a few words on the front of the package, like "natural" and "heart-healthy" are supposed to sell the product. Consumers who can't read a label that is written in scientific jargon default to the simple presentation on the front to know what they are buying. It is generally a false picture.

If you try to read a label for pastry dough it gets a lot worse with long complicated listings of multi-syllable words that, not only can you not pronounce them, but you would be hard pressed to find a reference for, even if you wanted to stay informed. Knowing that people hate to read small print, and that our technological age has produced many who no longer like to read, manufacturers try to make it as difficult as possible for consumers by longer and longer listings of huge words that have no meaning in common language.

Just a short word about language so you understand, if you don't speak the language where you are, you are totally dependent upon those who do. Refugees who escape to another country are often taken advantage of for that reason. Try communicating with those who are deaf and see what they think about how easy it is to communicate with those who can speak. Doctors and lawyers and other like professions have their own language, and it is often used to control others whether or not they look at it that way. Try leaving medical care if you don't agree with the diagnosis or treatment. They are offended if you leave.

If manufacturers can throw a new language at a population who are used to speaking one language, that of milk, eggs, sugar, and salt, what do you think the result will be? Yes, confusion and ignorance.

Let's back up for a minute. Think about **the physical** area in the context of health. It's the easiest one to examine since it can be perceived with our five senses, easier than, say, the emotions or mental states. Back in our history as a nation, physical health was simpler to maintain if you ignored accidents and battles. You were more likely to die being thrown by a horse, bit by a rattlesnake, or drowning in a river. You killed game, you collected nuts, seeds, and roots, and you grew your own vegetables. If you had a cow or goat, you had access to milk, butter, and cheese.

Physical health was balanced back then by the constant exercise and exertions that dominated life. You walked a lot. You felled trees and built your own buildings. You hiked long distances for game and carried the meat back home again. You maybe had a horse to make life a little easier. You hauled water. You chopped wood for heat. Lots of exercise, not like today.

Today we live what is called a sedentary lifestyle. Picture it! We sleep all night in a reclining position, we rise to maybe sit in a tub or stand in a shower, we sit at the table for breakfast, we sit in the car or on a bus to go to school or work, we sit all day in an office or at a desk unless we are fortunate enough to have a labor job, we sit for lunch, we sit in the car or on the bus going home, we sit and read the paper, or watch T.V., we sit at the table for dinner, sit some more until bedtime, then recline again for sleep. How much exercise do we see in that routine? Once a week maybe we mow the lawn unless we can pawn it off on one of our children or a neighbor boy.

With this lifestyle, there is nothing pumping fresh oxygen to our lungs, our blood lacks oxygen as do our brain cells. When we don't use our feet much, lymph does not circulate well to protect the body. Our feet are the pump. Our muscles atrophy to a certain extent. Our joints aren't used enough to lubricate themselves, so we are stiff and sore a lot. It's hard to get up out of a chair without feeling like a cripple. All those little knots of lactic acid in our muscle fibers don't break down properly without movement so our muscles ache daily.

The food we eat is next. Meat, potatoes, and vegetables can work well enough as healthy fare, but junk food is a huge problem. Did you know that, a long time ago, places that sold fast food used a study of colors to sell their junk food. The study suggested that the colors orange, yellow, red, and brown will start gastric juices flowing. Which businesses have you seen with some variation of those colors? So when we're driving down the street and our children spot the businesses using those colors, there is an instant request to stop and eat. Clever, huh?

Marketing techniques with food are endless, but have you noticed in walking down the cereal aisle in the grocery store how the sugar cereals are at the eye level of children and healthy cereals are on the top shelf. That way, our children can tug at our skirts or pant legs and ask us to buy them a certain cereal. Cartoons and prizes are attractive.

Restaurants serve ice water or coffee right away when we sit down because another study said that extremes in temperature will start gastric juices flowing. So, while we are perusing the menu, the hope is that the coffee we're sipping, or the ice water, will make us more hungry so that we order a bigger meal. Those working in a restaurant may not know why they serve you ice water and coffee, they just do what they're told, but there are executives who funded the study who know about it.

Labeling of foods is a real problem. The more we think we know what we're buying, the more corporations will work to confuse us. First, the label on a can or package was supposed to tell us exactly what was in it.

So, the label on a half-gallon of ice cream might say water, milk, sugar, flavoring. Supposedly putting labels on food was done because they used to put things like formaldehyde and kerosene in ice cream, just like they put cocaine in Coca Cola. The Safe Food and Drug Act of 1906 was a direct result of formaldehyde found in things like baby food and milk, and they were putting heroin in cough syrup. People wanted to know what they were actually getting. It was supposed to make the food companies be honest about their products.

The problem is that smaller companies who labeled their products truthfully were bought out by bigger companies, and bigger companies have the money for corporate lawyers and lobbyists in congress so they are able to overcome any resistance and swing the laws that are passed in their favor. Labels evolve. They still put harmful ingredients in products and food, they just label everything so it takes a chemist to decipher it. Nice guys!

If organic food, which is just simply food without chemicals, additives, toxins and other artificial ingredients, challenges commercial food in the super market, corporate lobbyists have watered down the organic laws so that using the organic label can mean 70% organic instead of 100%. If you think about it, thirty percent chemical and artificial ingredients is still a lot of fake stuff! You have to look for local, small business organic foods and farmer's markets to be safer. Stay away from national chains, except Costco, which is the only one I am aware of at this moment, which has declared a commitment to provide quality products that they have made public, and they have stocked many organic products.

Nowadays, labels you read are absolutely confusing, like we said earlier! Because of corporations swinging the laws in their favor again, they list scientific terms on a label. Instead of saying milk, sugar, and some kind of flavoring, now they say monocalcium phosphate, and thiamine mononitrate, and acesulfame potassium.

They have many different ways they can say sugar on a label. Let's say you are diabetic, or have a hyperactive child, or just like to watch your sugar intake. You have to learn to read labels. Besides saying sugar, they can also say sucrose, dextrose, dextrin, maltodextrin, corn syrup, high fructose corn syrup, monosaccharides, disaccharides, and sucralose, and they have synthetic sweetners whose names you couldn't pronounce. They could still add honey, agave, maple syrup, and molasses. If you are diabetic, it would be important to know this. Try being a single mother with a hyperactive child and trying to keep track of corporate shenanigans in labeling. What a headache!

I just reached in the cupboard and pulled out a box of prepackaged Apple Cider that says on the box "Sugar Free." The very first ingredient in the label, which everyone knows is the ingredient there is the most of, is maltodextrin! Who do they think they're fooling? Technically, when marketed products use maltodextrin they are extracting a sugar from malt instead of processing sugar beets or sugar cane, and so they want you to believe it isn't sugar. It has a similar effect on the body, though. Sugar is sugar in the body.

They have other names for salt, also, mainly called sodium something. They may have many sodium-somethings in one product. If you are on a low salt diet, it would be important to know that. Some sodium combinations are necessary but it would be good to know how much you're getting.

Everybody seems to like French fries. I like them, too, but they are an example of what we have been slowly doing to the foods we eat. You start with the potato, which in some circles is considered an almost perfect food by itself, having water, fiber, carbohydrates to burn, and most vitamins and minerals you would ever need, including vitamin C, the master vitamin.

For French fries, the potato is peeled of the part that has fiber, vitamins, and minerals. What you have left is starchy carbohydrates and water. The potato in this condition is sliced and dunked in boiling lard or cheap oil that cooks them quickly at high temperatures, a process studies tell us is carcinogenic. The carbohydrates soak up the oil, then salt is poured on them. You are served your plate of French fries stripped of all nutritional value, something that will some day contribute to your getting arteriosclerosis and high blood pressure, and they actually make you pay money for that! Yum!

There are other excesses with foods. Processed sugar is a pure poison and will do only harm to your system. White bleached flour and excessive caffeine are other culprits. Chemicals abound in foods where we used to exist just fine with zero chemicals in foods.

Some foods are not foods, now, with the advent of genetically modified products. Some foods have actually been synthesized in a laboratory, not grown in a garden or field, so that you could be served fake foods in restaurants now, or you might buy them in stores. There is even fake meat now that is used to make hamburgers and other products America holds dear.

Corporate America has seen to it that we can't even label foods GMO, or genetically modified, so you don't know sometimes what you're getting. Other countries have no trouble labeling GMO foods, but our country is still backward in that respect. Mostly GMO foods are corn, soy beans, wheat, and now even salmon, any food that can feed the masses efficiently. Those are the ones they are modifying first. Most European countries have banned GMO foods because they are believed to be harmful to human health.

So eating is an important step in the process of growing older. How do you think what you eat is affecting you in the long term? How much of old age grouchy behavior comes from being nutritionally deficient, do you think? Did you know that smoking will use up your levels of vitamin C and drinking will rob you of your B vitamins? Drugs will require many of your vitamins and minerals and they will give back heavy metals and other harmful chemical effects. Why do you think drug ads contain so many warnings about things?

I picked up a magazine in a doctor's office and saw a full-page ad promoting a drug in normal type, followed by two full pages of warnings about side effects and possible death written in small print. They finish off by advising you to ask your doctor, the one who doesn't have training in nutrition, if this drug is right for you. If you do your own thinking at all, you already know the answer to that question.

Without the right nutrition, cells can become abnormal. How much of what we consume brings us ever closer to that door of death we seem so afraid of?

I read where half of our mentally ill patients who were given doses of vitamin B12 were cured of mental illness and were able to return home again? That's back when they decided to release most of them into society again to become either homeless people or wards of social services.

Now we have a problem with obesity in America. Obesity is a common old age problem. What happens to a sheep or goat that eats the wrong plant? There is bloat that can be life-threatening. Their stomachs swell up. How much of the wrong foods do you think will cause our stomachs to bloat up?

If we go to cold climates, like Alaska, the body will store more fat for insulation. If we eat a lot of the wrong things, our bodies will store fat then, too, as a place to store toxins since toxins are stored in the fat of the body.

Exercise would move them as we burn fat so that toxins enter the blood stream and can be pumped out of the body by the heart, or so that toxins can leave the body through the sweat glands and pores. If we don't exercise, we just get fatter. More chemicals keep entering the body and they have to be stored somewhere. If not in fat, then in muscle and the body's organs.

Did you know that if we exercise, we burn fats first, then carbohydrates? If we sit watching T.V., we burn carbohydrates first.

Let me explain something about the colon. Colon cancer is one of our leading types of cancer in America. If we live a life of eating little fiber because we don't like fruits and vegetables and we eat white bread and Fruit Loops instead of whole grains, we will probably not have enough fiber in our systems to move waste along in the colon. We may also be constipated.

For a healthy colon, we need both fiber and water. Let's say we drink a lot of caffeine in teas, colas, and coffees, or we eat a lot of chocolate, which also has caffeine. Caffeine tells your body to get rid of water, called a diuretic. If what we need for a healthy colon is fiber and water, but we keep telling our bodies to lose water, while at the same time, we ignore fiber foods in our diets, like vegetables, what do we think will happen to our colons?

The walls of the colon undulate through a process called peristalsis. That undulation moves food along. The way it is supposed to work is that food enters the colon and lays there, water then swells the fiber in the food so both walls of the colon touch the food and move it along using peristalsis.

Have you ever seen a board that lays on grass for a length of time? If you lift it up, the grass is dying underneath, kind of a white color. That's what happens to colon cells when food lays there and isn't able to move along. Plus there are chemical reactions. Healthy cells can mutate to cancer cells. How many old people are constipated? That should tell you if you have enough fiber and water in your diet and whether or not you are getting enough exercise.

Now think about a poor diet, a poor exercise program, and on top of that you want to drink to excess, or smoke, or do drugs, or overeat, or maybe you want to cut yourself, or inhale things not good for you. If you treated a plant or animal how you treat yourself, how long do you think they would continue to live?

Risky behaviors is another category to consider in the area of health, the kind of "risky" that is impulsive. Some people drive fast, or they abuse someone else, or they put people at risk, as well as themselves, in other ways, like when the gas furnace filter is not maintained. Sometimes it's a simple thing, like when an uncle of mine spread chemical fertilizer with his bare hands without using gloves. A manly man doesn't need gloves, right? It killed him eventually. The chemicals were absorbed through his skin, affected his heart, he lost consciousness while driving.

There are so many ways we can hurt ourselves, it's really a wonder we make it to old age! Yet, there's something indomitable about the human spirit. It reminds me of the weeds at the side of the road that are mowed down, sprayed with chemicals, and covered with the salt solution we use on roads in the winter to melt ice. You will still see plants that we call weeds growing alongside the road, no matter what we do to them. Sometimes a lot of damage can be absorbed by a living thing, enough to sustain life.

If you consider that there are many circumstances in history where the proper diet has not been in place, and look at how many people survived it, it might let you see that food is a relative topic and it varies widely from individual to individual.

I mentioned ways to damage the body and be fooled by labels, but here's what is important to know. The average diet, if it is thoughtfully prepared, will be just fine when it comes to maintaining good health. There are exceptions, of course, when dealing with disease states or genetic abnormalities, even when dealing with the needs of special groups like newborns. But generally speaking, unless you are a junk food junkie or are living a life of deprivation, your diet will be fine for you.

Your body adjusts to your preferences and comfort foods, for the most part. The human body is very adept at managing variations and deprivations. It can handle a certain amount of damage and still function in a healthy way.

So, in spite of a gloomy picture involving corporate interference in our diets, realize that you have the power to control your own food. It just requires awareness and education. Read the latest articles and research and keep up with food changes. As you study the nutrients in food, like those newer minerals, see what they learn about them in future years. No matter what they learn, though, a good basic diet of fruits and vegetables, nuts, seeds, and whole grains, especially if they are organic, will serve you well.

Chapter 6 Acid/Base Balance

Approximately 20% of the diet needs of the body require acidic foods. The rest should be alkaline or a mixture of alkaline/acidic. The reason the acid/base balance is important to think about is the high incidence of junk foods, simple carbohydrates, and sugars in today's diet so that the food we consume is overly acidic. This leads to improper digestion and acidosis that will drain and weaken the health and energy of every cell in the body.

An alkaline diet is mostly vegetable or plant-based but there is more to it than that. Meat is listed as very acidic but meat is also rich in sulfur and phosphorus which are alkaline. There is a natural balance already in place with food. Besides, you would have to eat around 4 lbs. of lean meat in order to shift your body even slightly acidic.

Take the egg. Egg white is said to be nearly neutral, while egg yolks are very acidic. You will always get acid where you find proteins and fats. However, if you eat the whole egg together, white and yolk, the acidic level drops considerably to about 1/3. That is because there are balances built in.

Generally, we don't need to worry about acid-base balance with the average person. It is special circumstances that create the need to adjust diet. To explain briefly, the acid-base system in the body has several components that help maintain a balance. One is a system of **buffers** that do chemical work in the bloodstream. Secondly, there are the **lungs**, and thirdly, the **kidneys**. Consider this a crash course in pH balance.

The buffers are a bloodstream chemical-combining of acids and bases to make salts, which are alkaline. Most of the elements for this operation can be found in your food. Buffers hold pH at a constant level and resist any changes to the balance.

The lungs rid the body of the majority of acids through the respiration of CO_2, which is acidic. Those who have asthma, or those who smoke, those with sleep apnea have a special circumstance that might require an alteration in diet to correct an imbalance.

If you breathe hard, like with exercise, you create an alkaline environment. With exercise you also get lactic acid as a by-product, so it balances. If you snore or breathe heavy during sleep, thereby creating increased alkalinity, you quit breathing like with sleep apnea to build up CO_2 and restore a balance. There may be connections of a continual sleep apnea condition to the heart that are detrimental, but now you know why you stop breathing.

Holding your breath, shallow breathing (like with a sedentary lifestyle, i.e. watching T.V. or a lot or computer work), breathing CO_2 (like when hyperventilating and you breath into a paper bag), or if the heart is unable to adequately supply oxygen to the tissues, these create an acidic environment. So if a patient in the hospital is laying in bed sedentary and breathing shallow, they become acidic and sometimes they are given oxygen to increase the alkaline level of their blood.

People who smoke and damage their lungs are putting the body at a disadvantage when it comes to maintaining acid/base balance. Believe me, I have seen autopsied lung tissue from a smoker and the tissue is not pink, it is black, and it is full of large holes which make breathing increasingly more difficult. By the way, the lungs are an organ that can regenerate itself if a person stops smoking.

The kidneys are the third balancing system in the body and they regularly excrete acids. The reality of physiology is that the body continually produces acids, like in the oxidation of proteins and with CO_2 and with lactic acid from exercise, so the kidneys help us get rid of the excess.

Generally, the neutral point on pH is 7 and 7.4 is normal for most people. Lower than 6.9 leads to acidosis which has a final outcome of coma and death if acidosis is allowed to persist. Greater than 7.8 leads to alkalosis with a final outcome of convulsions and death if alkalosis is allowed to persist. So, this discussion is important! With the buffers, the lungs, and the kidneys, we have under normal conditions all we need to maintain a healthy acid/base balance.

You now have enough information to think through a specific situation to see if you think it requires adjustments in diet to restore pH balance. Normally you are fine, adjust only when certain special circumstances present themselves. Below are some foods that are alkaline so that you can plan meals and food purchases in the pursuit of correcting an imbalance. Remember moderation is a key! This is considered a temporary solution until balance is restored, if ever.

Litmus paper can be purchased so you can occasionally check the pH of your body. Test before a meal or when an hour has gone by after the meal. Testing is by mouth. If you test urine, since urine flushes acid, expect the results to be acidic.

Alkaline Foods

All green beans, all vegetables with spinach being the highest alkaline of them all by far, and tomato/V8 juices.

All fruits, juices, marmalade, nuts, and seeds except for peanuts and walnuts which are somewhat acidic. Raisins are considered the most alkaline by far.

Honey, sour cream, whole milk, egg white, yogurt, buttermilk, ice cream, wheat bread, rye crackers, white rice, lentils, peas, beans, butter, olive oil, soft cheeses, are all basically neutral, or being slightly acidic.

Draft beer, stout beer, cocoa, coffee, mineral water, wines, herb teas are alkaline. Just don't get carried away with the wine and the beer. Remember, temporary solution. I said *temporary!*

Chapter 7 Special Diets

People are different. You probably knew that. So are dietary needs. I have tried to give you an idea of diet versus nutrition in the following.

Allergies are usually solved by eliminating the offending food. The rest of the food group should be fine for offering nutrients. If a person has celiac disease, eliminating gluten means most grains are a problem, but nutrition is easily had by adding the other food groups. By *groups*, I mean meat, dairy, legumes, vegetables, fruits, nuts/seeds, and grains without gluten.

Those who are lactose intolerant can cut out dairy but find nutrients in the other groups. We're assuming here that people will seek a healthy diet. Allergies with shellfish leaves out the seafood group, and allergies to peanuts leaves out the nut group possibly, but the other groups make up the difference.

Low Salt diets require finding foods with low sodium, but sodium can be found in all food groups. Staying away from any processed food, which is high in sodium, is essential. Leaving the salt shaker in the cupboard, not on the table, is equally essential. Meats like fish and ham use salt as a preservative, cheese and butter have a lot of salt, and canned goods contain a lot of salt. High blood pressure is nothing to fool around with. It can be very damaging. Use good sense.

Most foods already have enough sodium naturally. However, if you're like my paternal grandmother, you add salt to water to make it boil quicker. You season foods as they cook. Then, at the table, you pick up the salt shaker and add more salt. That's a lot of salt!

In America, we use four things to flavor foods, one of which doesn't really harm you. Three of them, salt, fat, and sugar, are addictive and we go overboard in their use. It's the overboard that is harmful. Everything in moderation. The fourth thing is herbs and spices. Concentrate on those to flavor your foods.

Vegetarian/Vegan diets are a matter of finding food combinations that make a complete protein because, without meat and dairy protein, it is all that is left. These people must educate themselves on nutrition to stay healthy. Our bodies have a lot of good proteins doing very complicated jobs for us and proteins are in continual need of replacement and repair.

Beans and rice is an example of a complete protein and there are others already listed in this book. Still, without animal sources, this diet is deficient in nutrients like biotin unless eggs are an exception, vitamin B12 unless eggs or some dairy are exceptions, PABA is limited to the grain group, inositol needs to be supplemented, vitamin D is limited to the synthesis of sunshine on the skin, and cobalt needs to be supplemented.

All Protein diets I have heard of, which would mainly include the meat, dairy, legume, and nuts/seeds groups, but they require supplementation of other nutrients, like bioflavonoids, PABA unless you are willing to eat liver, silicon will have to come from legumes and almonds, iodine will come from

90

some dairy and iodized salt, and sulfur will have to be gotten from legumes and nuts/seeds. Too much protein is harmful and turns the body environment acidic, so acidosis is a real problem.

Diabetics, as is true with vegans, have to become mini-experts on the subject of dietary nutrition since, if they don't, there are dire consequences. This is a weight loss diet, smaller amounts that you then burn off through exercise, along with managing sugars and carbohydrates. There are plenty of books already on just this one subject alone. If this is your reality, I would suggest a good reference book be kept in your home that does more than generalize, as I am doing.

Raw Food is a concept I agree with philosophically but the modern human body, as it has physically developed, seems to need a percentage of cooked food also. I will repeat that raw food provides more vitamins while cooked food has more to offer with minerals.

The best information I could find in all of the sources used for this book was that the diet should have a 50/50 division of raw versus cooked food. So, fruit/vegetable snacks with nuts and seeds, and salads for raw. I have seen some very creative recipes in the raw food world that were delicious to eat, but for me, there wasn't enough variety. That's a personal preference. There are people who are more geared to this diet and thrive with it.

There are many special diets, like no sugar for hyperactivity, extra iron for iron-poor, anemic blood, pregnancy considerations when considering development of the fetus, the needs of children, the needs of the elderly, teenage requirements, and weight loss. These are individual needs and should be researched carefully for optimum health. No one book has all the answers, including this one. This book represents what I am able to find out so far, so the hope is that it will help educate you, then we'll see what future information pops up in further research to make you smarter.

Below are the food groups and **what nutrients are generally missing** if you only ate from that one group. This should help you make decisions since you can borrow from other food groups to get the proper balance of nutrients you need.

Missing Nutrients by Group

Meat: PABA, bioflavonoids, vitamin E, phosporus, copper, silicon, iodine (except seafood), sulfur. Liver has PABA and copper.

Dairy: PABA, vitamins A, C, K, bioflavonoids, selenium, silicon, fluorine, sulfur, molybdenum, strontium. Eggs have PABA and fluorine. Cheese has vitamin K.

Fruits: PABA, biotin, choline, vitamins B12 and D, inositol, copper, selenium, chromium, iodine, cobalt, chlorine, sulfur, molybdenum, strontium.

Vegetables: PABA, biotin, choline, vitamins B12 and D, inositol, copper, selenium, chromium, iodine unless you count seaweed, cobalt, fluorine, chlorine, strontium. You can get sulfur in beets, broccoli, and coconut. If you don't like those, you'd have to get sulfur somewhere else.

Legumes: PABA, bioflavonoids, biotin, vitamins B12, C, E, inositol, phosphorus, chromium, iodine, cobalt, flourine.

Nuts/Seeds: PABA, bioflavonoids, inositol, vitamins B12, C, D, K, chromium, silicon except for almonds, iodine, cobalt, fluorine except for pecans, chlorine.

Whole Grains: Vitamins A, B12, C, D, biotin, choline, bioflavonoids, inositol, silicon, iodine, cobalt, chlorine, sulfur. Flourine is only found in rice and oatmeal.

All Food Groups have vitamins B1, B2, niacin, B6, pantothenic acid, folacin, vitamin K, calcium, magnesium, iron, and manganese. Plus teas and coffees have bioflavonoids and antioxidant qualities, salt can be iodized, and water has chlorine. If you don't drink chlorinated water, and you are vegan, you may need to supplement.

Chapter 8 Basic Eating

I spent most of my life not liking salads, but habits and tastes sometimes have to change for good health. It's not that eating a different way, like I was, will kill you, but it can cause damage by depleting nutrients from other body processes.

Salad, if the proper food combinations are used, should contain no starch, like potatoes, no proteins, like eggs or shrimp, no oils, and no acids, like vinegar or lemon juice.

If you combine lettuces with tomatoes and cucumbers, that is the standard dinner salad in a restaurant. That's the salad I had trouble eating so I never ordered it.

To make salads more interesting, add to the standard salad things like fruits, nuts, berries, coconut, and seeds. I add tangerines, blueberries and raspberries, roasted pecans, sesame seeds, apples, cauliflower, broccoli, carrots, and avocado. Season these salads with pepper and herbs, if desired. There are other combinations that will work, also. This is where you are free to create. If you have enough stuff in a salad, there is always plenty of taste.

Nuts are a protein food, technically, but I make an exception for them because of personal preference. You can make small exceptions for the sake of happiness. In this case, tomatoes help offset an undesirable result from the combination. The same is true if cottage cheese is used, which is also a protein food. Use tomatoes with it.

It can also make a tasty salad if pickled things are added, like beets, 4-bean type, artichoke hearts, asparagus, or olives. These also go well with cottage cheese plain or with the lettuce salad. I make exceptions for minor additions as is true of 4-bean salad, they add a little sweetener, or artichoke hearts which have an oil, but everything in moderation, right? You won't die because you made an exception in a normal diet.

A salad that has this many ingredients will have a naturally pleasant taste and will not need dressings, however, if you need something, try olive oil as a dressing since it has many health benefits. Just know that nuts and oil are not good together.

A fruit salad is sweeter and can be topped off with fresh lime juice, also adding nuts and seeds, coconut, and avocado if desired. Salads should be eaten separately, not with protein and starch, so I eat mine a half-hour before the other foods if they are still cooking, or a half-hour after for desert. A half-hour-or-so separation is enough time. The same is true of fruit. A half-hour separation from other foods is best. Eat a fruit as a snack or a dessert.

Acid fruits do not combine well with sweet fruits. Green vegetables do not combine well with sweet fruits. Protein, starch, and fat do not combine well with sweet fruits. Melons do not combine well with either sweet or acid fruits.

Sugar, like in whipped cream, molasses, agave, honey, and syrup, combine badly with all foods and are best when not eaten in combination, or not eaten at all. We learned to use them to sweeten bland foods in pioneer days when varieties of food items were scarce, but sugar is in everything now and we get an overabundance of it in the body. This forms an acidic environment that is detrimental to the human body.

If you use exceptions here, use local honey or a product like Stevia, occasionally 100% maple syrup. In a recipe, instead of sugar, substitute half the amount of honey. Honey is more concentrated so you need less of it.

Processed sugar acts as a poison and has no nutritional value. Over time, people start showing signs of poisoning, like bloating, stomachs that we can't get rid of. Poisoning by processed sugar, over-consumption of alcohol, consuming chemicals and other toxins cause us to become fatter to build storage for toxins.

After salads, think soup. Soups are excellent for health because they provide water, vegetables with their nutrients and fiber, whole grains if you add barley, rice, and ancient grains, with their nutrients and fiber, beans and lentils with their high fiber, and meat if you are not vegetarian or vegan. In addition, when foods are heated in water, the exchange of nutrients from food to water stays as a healthy broth when it is in a soup.

Soups are low calorie meals, as are salads. If no bread or crackers are consumed with these meals, the calories stay low. Adding bread or crackers is an individual choice when considering body weight. There are many whole grain, low salt, even gluten-free bread or cracker varieties, in that case.

With meats, sticking to low fat varieties is healthy, so fish, chicken, turkey. I buy only organic meats. If you need some red meat, try a lean organic hamburger for fixing meat balls, meat loaf, lasagna, spaghetti sauce, and so forth. Remember to eat smaller amounts of food, especially if you are sedentary. It may work to use the small plates for your meal.

Athletes need more protein than others, and since exercise breaks down cholesterol, red meats are usually okay for them. The problem comes in when they stop being athletes but they have eating habits that are not adjusted to retirement from sports. Weight gain is inevitable, cholesterol build-up, and other problems creep in.

If an athlete is vegetarian, food combinations need special attention to get enough protein for muscle building and repair. There are cases of vegetarian athletes who continually broke bones and tore ligaments because of this.

Remember advice like "never eat until you are full," and "chew your food carefully" so that digestive enzymes in your saliva have a chance to mix with the food and begin breaking it down. Digestion begins in the mouth. Also, "grow your own food," and "use distraction to avoid eating too many times."

Distractions keep you busy so you don't obsess on eating. Get a hobby or begin a project. If you are landscaping the yard or cutting quilt squares, you are not eating or thinking about eating. Distraction will help until your stomach adjusts to longer times between meals and smaller amounts. Your stomach will adjust. Be confident.

Restaurants use salt, sugar, and fats to flavor foods, so eat out sparingly. Everything in moderation. They also, generally speaking, don't pay attention to things like chemicals in the food, GMO's, lab-created food, factory farming, and sanitation standards are up to the individual restaurant. In a restaurant you tend to over-eat. You accept white flour, sugars, caffeine, alcohol, and other conditions much more readily. You will have to spend several days trying to balance the body again after making these exceptions to your normal diet. As always, as a thinker, choose wisely.

Those who desire sandwich-type foods may benefit from what we do in my house, which is to use Romaine lettuce leaves as bread, wrapping wild salmon salad, or guacamole, or refried beans, or cheeses in them with fresh, chopped tomato. These are good for diabetic diets and for those seeking low-calorie meals. Or you may want to switch to tortillas, pita bread, or nan, the Indian bread.

The ingredients you use are many and varied if you are creative. Meat eaters can reduce the amount of food consumed during a meal by making a meat loaf that also contains things like onions, whole grain bread crumbs, eggs, greens such as spinach, ground flax, seeds, chopped mushrooms, and any number of other ingredients. It is possible to cover all of the food groups if topped with a mango salsa, which is a delicious substitute for ketchup which contains sugar. You are only limited by your imagination.

Approaching food according to the nutrients that can make you healthy can be a creative process. That makes what you do in the kitchen a work of art, and art inspires any artist. Preparing food does not have to be a chore.

Chapter 9 Pregnancy

First of all, a 25 lb. to 30 lb. weight gain during pregnancy is healthy. If a woman starts her pregnancy underweight, then perhaps she needs a 28-40 lb. weight range. Overweight women are often encouraged to gain 15-25 lbs. during pregnancy.

To support fetal growth, extra amounts of nearly all nutrients are required in the diet. A vitamin and mineral supplement is often recommended. There must also be abstinence from alcohol, and a limited intake of caffeine, the equivalent of two cups of coffee per day.

Calories

Approximately 2400-2600 calories per day to support a pregnancy using mostly fruits and vegetables, whole grains, lean meats, and legumes, with nuts and seeds, olive or coconut oils, and dairy.

Allow for a 14-ounce weight gain per week during the last 30 weeks of pregnancy. Much is individual, like how much exercise one gets, and so forth.

Protein

Extra protein will be required during pregnancy, approximately 60 g/day total.

Fat

No more than 30% of calories as fat. This is true for everyone. Foods containing omega-3 fats are best for fetal development of brain and nerve tissue.

Exercise

Yes, please do exercise. Just keep your chosen exercise from stressing you.

Vitamins and Minerals for Pregnancy

Folic acid is needed for fetal neural function; *vitamin B12* for synthesis of fetal blood; *thiamine, riboflavin, and niacin* for production of energy for the mother; *vitamin B6* for fetal protein synthesis, and to reduce nausea, vomiting, depression in the mother; *iron* for fetal hemoglobin in red blood cells, sometimes needs supplement; *zinc* to boost enzyme function; *magnesium* to support fetal and maternal tissue growth; *iodine* to avoid physical and developmental delays in the fetus; *calcium* for skeletal development in the fetus, to prevent hypertension in the mother; *biotin* for breast-feeding; **pantothenic acid** for optimum health; *water* always because fluid needs for both mom and fetus increase dramatically during pregnancy.

Water and fiber are both needed to combat a common pregnancy problem, that of course is constipation, caused by pressure exerted on the intestines by the enlarging uterus, mineral supplements, and/or decreasing of physical activity.

It is important not to be deficient in the vitamins and minerals listed above, as birth defects have been associated with deficiencies. Try to get most, if not all, of food nutrients from your daily meals, if possible. If not, supplement carefully since it doesn't take much of an overdose to stress a fetus.

Food Cravings

We have all heard the pickles and ice cream stories during pregnancy, but there are times when tastes lead people to eat things like clay or other non-food items, a condition called pica. Just be careful not to substitute cravings for a wholesome diet, and be careful the cravings aren't dramatically altering calorie count. Diabetes can become a problem during pregnancy. Be aware. Keep sugar and carbohydrates to an absolute minimum.

Eating smaller, more frequent meals is better with a shrinking stomach, and being upright after eating helps with acid reflux. Sitting in a straight-backed chair helps with backache. Carrying a larger stomach, just like men with potbellies, can stress the lower back, so soak in a tub, use a hot-water bottle, get a loving husband to massage you, use back support like weight-lifters do.

Vegetarian/Vegan Women
Take extra care to be sure the above listed vitamins and minerals are in good supply in the diet, including protein combinations.

Chapter 10 Foods That Detox

Toxins, free radicals, and other potentially harmful substances need to be flushed from the body. The bulk of this detoxing work is accomplished by the lymph system, the liver, and the kidneys. To keep them from toxic overloads, it is important to reduce chemicals in foods by buying organic. Organic presently costs more, but you need less of those foods because they are concentrated, so less cost overall. You can easily eat smaller amounts to stay healthy and lose weight, where the same cannot be said of food that is not organic. That food is cheaper at first but will increase the toxin load for your body systems. The cheaper foods will cost you far more in the long run in health care problems that develop from being nutrient deficient.

To help out, there are certain foods, while not magic potions, that will help you in the process of detoxing the body. They are the following, in alphabetical order.

Artichokes
Helps the liver to function well, plus contains fiber, protein, magnesium, folate, and potassium.

Asparagus
Helps to detox, helps as anti-aging agent, helps protect against cancer, anti-inflammatory, and heart healthy.

Avocado
Contains healthy fat, is an antioxidant, and good fiber.

Beets
Help make sure toxins actually make it out of the body, they are an anti-cancer aid, a super food.

Broccoli
Packs a nutritional punch, specifically works with enzymes in the liver to transform toxins into that which can be eliminated from the body, but *do not microwave.*

Cabbage
Helps to cleanse the liver and lowers cholesterol, helps you go to the bathroom, which in turn eliminates toxins.

Dandelions
Dandelion root has several healing properties for the liver, strengthening and cleansing it.

Garlic
Helps the liver, boosts the immune system, adds taste to other detoxing foods, can be taken as supplement.

Ginger
Helps the liver, has astringent properties, especially for overconsumption of alcohol.

Grapefruit
Fiber, nutrient rich, detox punch, floods the body with good things while dislodging bad things, good for weight loss since it makes the liver burn up fat, kick-starts the liver for detoxing.

Green Tea
High antioxidant properties which seeks out and kills free radicals, a beverage that benefits the body.

Kale
Nutrient rich, flushes kidneys, fights kidney disease, antioxidant, anti-inflammatory.

Lemongrass
Helps liver and kidneys, as well as the bladder and the entire digestive tract and circulatory system.

Lemon
Flushes toxins from the body, helps with digestion.

Olive Oil
Triggers liver to get rid of gallstones, your go-to oil for eating raw foods, helps with elimination.

Seaweed/Kelp
Tons of nutrients, antioxidant, good detox food.

Turmeric
Beneficial to liver, can drink turmeric tea for a week to detox without any other detox foods.

Water
Flushes toxins, aids kidney function, carries toxins out of body through elimination, sweat, and tears.

Watercress

Along with cilantro and parsley, boosts the liver by releasing enzymes that get rid of toxic build-up, attaches to heavy metals and leads them out of the body.

Wheatgrass

Great boost to liver, alkaline, lowers blood sugar, gets metabolism back on track.

Five things to avoid:

1) alcohol,
2) processed flour and sugar as well as any other processed foods,
3) caffeinated beverages
4) sweets, candies, chocolates
5) overeating

All of this advice is tempered with common sense and moderation, of course. Fat chance you'll give up things like wine or chocolate, but remember, moderation in all things. These "don'ts" have mostly to do with not adding more toxins to your diet.

Note: Pesticides, herbicides, fungicides, insecticides are being sprayed on or around everything in our environment and they can cause such common symptoms as headaches and upset stomach, such unusual symptoms as tinnitus and vertigo, and such dangerous symptoms as seizures and body organ damage, not to mention death. Children and fetal development are especially vulnerable. Our bodies will store a certain amount before there is a toxic overload. Detoxing the body systems is an important consideration.

Chapter 11 Food Allergies

When I was a kid, you hardly ever heard the term "food allergy." I didn't know anyone who was allergic to anything. Now, it seems, everyone is. The human body is designed to be healthy. The body itself has not changed since I was a little kid, so logically speaking, the difference has to be the environment.

There are generally half-a-dozen factors that could affect the health of our bodies:

    a. genetic factors

    b. stress

    c. the lack of proper sleep

    d. physical trauma

    e. the lack of proper nutrients, and

    f. toxins (including radiation and GMO's)

There are over 2,000 additional chemical compounds that are approved for use each year in the United States, most of which do not exist in nature. Our bodies try to eliminate them but the burden of toxins is great.

When I was a kid, you didn't hear of cancer except lung cancer and leukemia. Our number one cancer now is colon cancer but you didn't hear of it back then. You also didn't hear of immune compromises like lupus, rheumatoid arthritis, Fibromyalgia, chronic fatigue syndrome, and other autoimmune diseases. You didn't hear of autism, or hyperactivity, or Alzheimers.

Until almost 1950, the diseases that were our top killers were related to bacteria and viruses, things like tuberculosis and pneumonia, things we couldn't see and didn't know existed until the advent of the microscope, and the discovery of penicillin in 1947. Now our top killers are called "lifestyle" diseases. Cancer, heart disease, diabetes, stroke are all lifestyle-related. That means we have control over them.

The areas we use to prevent lifestyle diseases are **diet**, **exercise**, **rest**, and **peace of mind**. These areas cover the physical, emotional, mental, and spiritual health of all human life. We have control over what we eat, what we think, how much exercise we get, and how much rest we get. The object of this book is to give control back to the average person using latest information.

Our grandparents ate real, seasonal foods from the farm, they didn't diet or limit what they ate, they cooked their own food from scratch, they had no preservatives, artificial ingredients, additives, GMO's, or chemical toxins in their food, they ate the whole animal, including boiling down bones and using organ meats, they walked a lot more, and they spent lots of time outside.

Believe it or not, they didn't go to the doctor when they got sick, rather relying on home remedies, and they didn't take prescription drugs. They saved doctor visits for things like accidents. They saved dental visits for things like a sore tooth.

Allergies, being a relatively new problem, are happening because of the environment. Gluten-free is here because wheat is one of the most chemicalized grains, along with soy and corn. Corn is a problem for some because it is chemicalized and GMO. Soy is rumored to be next for GMO, and who knows after that.

There are lactose-intolerant people because we kill the digestive enzyme in milk when raw milk is submitted to high temperatures in pasteurizing. The whole country used to be on raw milk with no sickness, it was taught as a whole food in school, and it was considered to be the healthiest food for everyone. Now it is against the law. Why?

Louis Pasteur developed the process of pasteurization to meet the demands of a disease out of control at the time, but even he was against using pasteurization as a cure-all and recommended it be used on a temporary basis to solve an immediate disease threat.

There are actual allergies that need medical intervention, but many allergies have been created by the food industry because of the way they process food, and by agricultural chemicals that are sprayed on our food supply.

Regardless, children with allergies need our attention since they live our lifestyle. Some common signs of allergies in children are frequent runny nose, dry skin patches on the face, especially around the mouth, stuffy sinuses, dark bags and possibly swelled bags under the eyes, and a horizontal line across the tip of the nose where the bone stops. They try to breathe easier, so push their nose up often and it makes a permanent line.

Seeing an allergy specialist can help identify what foods are involved, but those without medical coverage will find testing expensive. You can conduct your own test by adding and eliminating foods until you see a relationship of a food to the symptoms your child has. With children, you might also suspect pollens or chemicals where they play, and reactions to vaccinations. If your husband sprays chemicals on the lawn and your children then play on the grass, ...you see? You have to become a thinking person.

Chapter 12 Super Foods

Super foods are so-called because they are the foods with the most nutrients and the least negative properties, like salt and fats. They are whole foods that work together in a basic healthy diet. From these as your core, you can add in things like bacon and chocolate as you choose.

Beans – fiber, iron, folate, B vitamins, potassium, magnesium

Blueberries – carotenoids, fiber, folate, vitamins C & E, potassium, magnesium, manganese, iron, riboflavin, niacin

Broccoli – folate, fiber, calcium, vitamins C & K, iron, beta-carotine

Flaxseed – omega3 fatty acids, fiber, protein, magnesium, iron, potassium

Oats – high fiber, protein, low calories, magnesium, potassium, zinc, copper, manganese, selenium, thiamine

Oranges – fiber, vitamin C, folate, potassium

Pumpkin (carrots & squash) – alpha carotene, beta carotene, high fiber, low calories, vitamins C & E, potassium, magnesium, pantothenic acid

Spinach – beta carotene, low calories, omega 3, vitamins C, E, B, calcium, zinc, magnesium, iron, manganese

Soy – omega 3, vitamin E, potassium, folate, magnesium, selenium, protein

Tea – flavanoids, fluoride, 0 calories, supports heart health by lowering LDL's

Tomatoes – vitamins C, B, A, beta carotene, low calories, potassium, chromium, biotin, fiber

Turkey (skinless breast) – protein, low fat, niacin, vitamins B6 & B12, iron, selenium, zinc

Walnuts – omega 3, vitamins E & B6, magnesium, protein, fiber, potassium

Wheat Germ – low calories, protein, fiber, folate, thiamine, manganese, vitamin E & B6, selenium, potassium, iron, zinc, omega 3

Wild Salmon – omega 3, selenium, potassium, protein, vitamins B & D

Yogurt – active cultures, complete protein, calcium, potassium, magnesium, zinc, vitamins B2 & B12, probiotics

Interchangeable Support (family) Groups

Grains with wheat germ and wheat bran

Beans with other beans, peas, lentils

Blueberries with other berries, cherries

Broccoli with brussel sprouts, kale, cabbage, turnips, cauliflower, collard and mustard greens, chard, bok choy

Oats with other grains

Oranges with lemons, grapefruit, kumquats, tangerines, limes

Pumpkin with carrots, squash, sweet potatoes, orange bell pepper

Salmon with halibut, tuna, sardines, herring, trout, sea bass, oysters, clams

Soy with tofu, soymilk, soy nuts, edamane, tempeh, miso

Spinach with kale, collards, chard, mustard/ turnip and beet greens, bok choy, romaine, orange bell pepper

Yogurt with kefir

Walnuts with other nuts

Turkey with skinless chicken breast

Tomatoes with red watermelon, pink grapefruit, red persimmon, red papaya, strawberry guava

Chapter 13 Weight Loss

I'll make it brief. You need an all-around basic nutrient-rich diet. Don't skimp or skip on that part. Losing weight, unless there is a genetic component or disease state, is largely a matter of eating less and exercising more. Eat fewer calories, burn more calories. When you exercise, you burn fat first.

Exercise pumps oxygen to every cell in the body along with the vitality each cell needs. Exercise breaks down cholesterol, helps keep blood pressure even, and pumps lymph where it needs to go. The whole body is revitalized, so you can't avoid exercise.

We're not talking going out for sports here, nor do we mean calisthenics. Simple walking every day is enough. If you don't go out, walk the stairs, or walk around the house or the yard. Bend over and pick up things. If you don't move, you get stiff and sore. Dust. Mop. Sweep the house, then the sidewalk in front of your house. Pull weeds. Carry the laundry. Or carry kids. Load-bearing exercise helps build bone and stave off osteoporosis. Carry groceries from the car. Rake leaves. Aerobics.

There are many things we can do to help ourselves. Substitute small snacks for large meals. Use the smaller plates. Determine to stick to one helping. No dessert unless maybe fruit or yogurt. If you really have a lot of weight to lose, try three grapes for dessert. Get creative, but find the balance between calories in and calories burned. Forget other diets unless for high blood pressure, diabetes, and other conditions that are prescribed for you. Lose weight by being sensible.

Chapter 14 Understanding Germs

For all of recorded history germs and viruses caused disease, but since they were invisible we blamed disease on sinful behavior, the devil, an angry god, and other such ways of thinking. Since germs were finally discovered, it was thought that if you eliminated germs altogether, you also eliminated disease altogether. The trouble with that was that extremes in sanitation made one even more susceptible to germs when they appeared. No immunity.

Extreme sanitation works in an operating room, or in a restaurant, and here's why. To put it simply, my germs are not your germs. America's germs are not the germs of Africa. The germs in town are not the germs of a rural farm.

We use sanitation when serving someone who is not from our area, or from our immediate environment. We use it for hospital patients, for guests, for different cultures, and so forth. We probably are safe enough in the same family who share germs. Safe enough in the same army outfit that shares environment, but they may not be safe in the environment of a foreign country. That's why we vaccinate.

In a family, a new baby learns immunity through slight sicknesses that build strength as the body fights them off. In a daycare or school, the same baby can become deathly ill because of the germs of other kids.

Dirt has minerals and other benefits, ask any farmer, but dirt can hold other surprises. Your dirt is okay for you, maybe not for me. We wash hands before handling food as a precaution to keep everybody safe.

Chapter 15 Emotions

Emotions affect food, which affects the way it is processed in your body. This has been well-known for centuries but we have not given it any importance in education.

We already know that emotions can have an adverse effect on everything, when we lose our temper, when we create dramas, when we are so depressed that we consider suicide an option. Food is affected by these, too. Food is energy on the atomic level. *We* are energy on the atomic level. Just like when we cook and food molecules exchange with the molecules of the pan or water, our emotional energy will exchange with the energy of food.

When we prepare food, it should be with happy love in our hearts for the wonderful abundance that is ours. This is the reason for a prayer before eating, also. It is a positive, thankful, energy exchange with the food we consume, then it can do its best work for us when we eat it.

If you are upset, fighting, or frustrated while preparing food, a different exchange takes place that has an end-result of the food being passed through the body without being used. Body cells actually change their electromagnetic polarity which causes this to happen.

Many relatively bad things can happen as we live life in this world, but those things build strength if we survive them. Our job is to find our happy place. We have to concentrate on finding joy and peace in the fact that all we have experienced has led us to where we are now so that a new beginning is possible. Then our food will help us to be healthy.

Chapter 16 Final Thoughts

Experiments were conducted at one time to see what would happen if you let babies, who were already on solid food, choose their own foods. Selections of different foods were laid out within their reach and they chose foods according to their whims. It was kind of an interesting study!

It was known that animals had an instinct for selecting a balanced diet if they were free to choose their own food, but the current belief was that humans lacked that instinct. The study involving babies hoped to clear up the question.

As it turned out, over a week's time, the babies were able to easily choose a balanced diet since they had not yet been conditioned to accept or reject foods based on prejudices or taste. We who have had children know that babies will put virtually anything in their mouths as a way of experimenting with their world. These babies didn't just eat what tasted pleasant, but they tasted everything and chose what was good for them without prompting, even if the taste was bland, bitter, or sour. By now, in adulthood, we have placed our food preferences in cement and it is darned hard to change them. We easily turn our noses up at foods we aren't used to and hold tightly to our poor eating habits.

One other thing, there are certain adult groups who have made a conscious decision to eliminate animal products from their diets based on moral objections regarding the killing of animals, but they haven't made that choice by instinct, nor have they made the choice because of holding tightly to poor eating habits. Having made what they feel is an informed decision, they now have to review the physiology of the body to ensure their future good health.

So many things in the human body are composed of the amino acids that make up protein that, if our chief source of protein, animal protein, is not acceptable, protein has to come from plant sources. It takes work to find combinations that provide enough amino acids to benefit the body. Some people aren't aware of how important it is to be educated on this subject.

Without enough protein, as is usually the case in the undernourished, the body will literally feed on itself, on the stores of fats and proteins we have until enough fuel comes again from food. In this case, the body shrinks to a degree as with the elderly, muscles shrink, cells give up their protein linings and the fluid that escapes becomes what we call edema (swelling) in the lower extremities usually. An example of a protein is the hemoglobin in your blood. Also, the heart and your other organs. Enzymes and hormones, too. All proteins important to health. Enough protein has to be taken into the body from the diet to perform maintenance and repair to keep the body in good shape.

You have probably seen the pictures of starving children who have pot-bellies and you might be tempted to think they don't really look starved with a belly like that. The protein lining around the cells is one of the very last things to go during starvation. The condition of the bellies has to do with edema, the fluid that has escaped the cells when the lining is gone. It collects and creates a pot-belly, one of the last stages before death.

Addenda

Addendum A
Handy Graph Information

Common Food Additives

Here are some of the many scientific words we can get brain fog from. Their role in storing food is outlined to eliminate some of the mystery while you are label-reading to aid you in decision-making.

PH Control
Acetic acid
Apidic acid
Citric acid
Lactic acid
Phosphates
Phosphoric acid
Sodium acetate
Sodium citrate
Tartaric acid

Mat/Bleach/Condit
acetone peroxide
azodicarbonamide
benzoyl peroxide
calcium bromate
potassium bromate
sodium stearyl fumarate
(mat/bleach/condit refers to maturing and bleaching agents and dough conditioners)

Stabil/thick/tex
Ammonium alginate
Arabinogalactan
Calcium alginate
Carob bean gum
Carrageenan
Cellulose
Gelatin
Guar gum
Gum Arabic
Gum ghatti
Karaya gum
Larch gum
Locust bean gum
Mannitol
Modified food starch
Pectin
Potassium alginate
Potassium bromate
Propylene glycol

Color
annatto extract
beta-apo-8'carotenal
beta-carotene
canthaxanthin
caramel
carrot oil
citrus Red #2
cochineal extract
corn endosperm
dehydrated beets
dried algae meal
Blue #1
Red #3
Red #40
Yellow #5
grape skin extract
iron oxide
paprika
riboflavin

125

Stabil/thick/tex (con't).
Sodium alginate
Sodium calcium alginate
Tragacanth gum
(stabil/thick/tex refers to
Stabilizers, thickners,
And texturizers)

Color (con't.)
saffron
tagetes (Aztec Marigold)
titanium dioxide
Turmeric
Ultramarine Blue

Nutrient
Ascorbic acid
Beta-carotene
Iodine
Iron
Niacinamide (niacin)
Potassium iodide
Riboflavin
Thiamin
Tocopherols (vitamin E)
Vitamin A
Vitamin C (ascorbic acid)
Vitamin D (vitamin D2, D3)

Antioxidant
ascorbic acid
BHA
BHT
citric acid
EDTA
propyl gallate
tocopherols (vit. E)
vitamin C

Leavening
calcium phosphate
Sodium alum. sulfate
sodium bicarbonate

Preservative
Ascorbic acid (vit. C)
Benzoic acid
Butylparaben
Calcium lactate
Calcium sorbate
Citric acid
Heptylparaben
Lactic acid
Methylparaben
Potassium propionate
Potassium sorbate
Propionic acid
Propylparaben
Sodium benzoate
Sodium diacetate
Sodium arythorbate
Sodium nitrate
Sodium propionate
sodium sorbate
sorbic acid

Anticaking
calcium silicate
iron ammonium citrate
mannitol
silicon dioxide
yellow prussiate of soda

Emulsifier
carrageenan
digycerides
dioctyl sodium sulfosuccinate
lecithin
monogycerides
polysorbates
sorbitan monostearate

Flavor Enhancer
Disodium guanylate
Disodium inosinate
Hydrolyzed vegetable protein
MSG (monosodium glutamate)
Yeast-malt sprout extract

Humectant (helps retain moisture)
Glycerine
Glycerole monostearate
Propylene glycol
Sorbitol

Flavor
Paprika
Spices
Turmeric (oleoresin)
Vanilla

Sweetners
Corn syrup
Dextrose
Sucrose
Fructose
Glucose
Invert sugar
Mannitol
Saccharin
Sorbitol

Addendum B
Conversion Tables

Length

USA	Metric
Inch	= 2.54 cm or 25.4 mm
Foot	= 0.30 m or 30.48 cm
Yard	= 0.91 m or 91.4 cm
Mile (statute)	= 1.61 km or 1609 m
(5280 ft.)	
Mile (nautical)	+ 1.85 km or 1850 m
(6077 ft.)	
(1.15 statute miles)	

Metric	USA
Millimeter	= 0.039 in.
Centimeter	= 0.39 in.
Meter	= 3.28 ft. or 39.37 in.
Kilometer	= 0.62 miles

Weight

USA	Metric
Grain	= 64.80 mg
Ounce	= 28.35 g
Pound	= 453.60 g or 0.45 kg
Ton (short – 2000 lbs.)	= 0.91 metric ton or 907 kg

Metric	USA
Milligram	= 0.002 grain or .000035 oz.
Gram	= 0.04 oz.
Kilogram	= 35.27 oz. or 2.20 lbs.
Metric ton (1000 kg)	= 1.10 tons

Volume

USA	Metric
Cubic inch	= 16.39 cc
Cubic foot	= 0.03 m (cubed)
Cubic yard	= 0.765 m (cubed)

Volume (con't.)

USA	Metric
Ounce	= 0.03 liters or 30 ml
Pint	= 0.47 liters
Quart	= 0.95 liters
Gallon	= 3.79 liters

Metric	USA
Milliliter	= 0.03 oz.
Liter	= 2.12 pt.
Liter	= 1.06 qt.
Liter	= 0.27 gal.

Note: 1 ml =1 cc

Formulas for converting temperature:

Degrees C = (degrees F – 32) x 5/9

Degrees F = 9/5 x (degrees C) + 32

-40 degrees F = -40 degrees C
32 degrees F = 0 degrees C
98 degrees F = 37 degrees C
212 degrees F = 100 degrees C

Simple Math

A **gram** is about 1/30th of an ounce (28 grams to the ounce)

5 grams is about 1 teaspoon

A **kilogram** is 1000 grams, equivalent to 2.2 pounds

A **pound** weighs 454 grams

A gram can be divided into 1000 **milligrams** (mg) or 1,000,000 **micrograms** (mcg)

Liters are almost equal to 1 quart or 4 cups

There are 3 teaspoons per tablespoon
16 tablespoons per cup
2 cups to a pint
2 pints or 4 cups to a quart
4 quarts to a gallon
16 ounces to a pound

Each day we need about 1 pound or 500 grams of energy-yielding substances in the food we eat. Add to this about 5 pounds of water. Aside from water, food is mostly a mixture of proteins, carbohydrates, and fats. You need some of each group for good health.

Addendum C
Body Systems at a Glance

Digestive System
> Mouth – teeth grind food, digestive enzymes in saliva
> Esophagus – food transport
> Stomach – stomach acid breaks down food
> Small intestine – enzymes from intestinal wall, from
> the pancreas, and bile from the liver mix with
> food and nutrients are extracted and sent where
> they can contribute to the health of the body
> Large intestine – elimination of what doesn't get
> absorbed

Skeletal System
> Bones, Joints, Muscles, Connective tissue

Nervous System
> Brain, Spinal Cord, Nerves

Circulatory System
> Blood, Blood Vessels, Heart

Respiratory System
> Nose, Trachea, Lungs

Urinary System
> Kidneys, Bladder, Urethra, Genitals

Endocrine System
> Pituitary Gland, Thyroid Gland, Parathyroid Glands,
> Pancreas, Adrenal Glands, Ovaries, Testes, Pineal
> Gland, Placenta

Immune System
> Lymph, Spleen, Tonsils, Thymus, Skin, Intestinal
> Walls, White Blood Cells

Addendum D
The Endocrine System

Pituitary Gland
Stores hormones secreted by the hypothalamus:
1. **oxytocin** (pitocin) – stimulates the uterus to contract at childbirth, maintains labor, and Influences the lactating breast to release milk
2. **vasopressin** (pitressin) (ADH) – antidiuretic; increases arterial pressure and enhances reabsorption of water
3. produces hormones that control the activity of a number of endocrine glands
4. produces growth hormone, instrumental in protein, fat, carbohydrate metabolism; located in the brain

Thyroid Gland
Produces the hormone **thyroxine**, which functions in at least 20 different enzyme systems and regulates the speed of virtually all of the basic cellular processes of the body; located at the base of the throat

Parathyroid Glands
There are usually four located near the thyroid which excrete a hormone, the **parathyroid hormone**, that has an important regulating effect on calcium and phosphorus

Thymus Gland
Located behind the sternum (chest area) and important in development of immune response in the newborn and in the manufacture of lymphocytes

Pancreas
Synthesis, storage, and secretion of **insulin**, which regulates the cellular uptake of sugar and blood sugar level; located below the heart

Stomach
Produces **gastrin** which stimulates secretion of stomach acid

Endocrine System (con't.)

Adrenal Glands

One superior to each kidney, which secretes:

Mineralocorticoids (aldosterone) which regulate sodium retention and supports electrolyte metabolism

Glucocorticoids (cortisol) which influence the metabolism of protein, fat, and glucose (carbs)

Androgens (testosterone) steroid hormones that produce masculinity

Ovaries

Produce two hormones:

Estrogen responsible for growth of female figure and organs, development of sexual characteristics, support of menstruation and ovulation

Progesterone maintains development of placenta, supports pregnancy and lactation

Testes

Produces **testosterone**, which supports proliferation of sperm and male sexual systems

Pineal Gland

Found in the middle of the brain; site of melatonin synthesis

Placenta

Produces **chorionic gonadotropin**, a hormone that stimulates the gonads, **estrogen**, and **progesterone**

Addendum E
Vitamins/Minerals Help

Bones – A, C, D, calcium, magnesium, phosphorus, zinc, silicon, manganese, fluorine,, strontium

Teeth – A, B6, C, E, pantothenic acid, calcium, phosphorus, fluorine, molybdenum, strontium

Skin – A, B2, B6, E, niacin, biotin, PABA, inositol, bioflavonoid, zinc

pH Balance – sulfur, chlorine, sodium, potassium

Vision – A, B2, C, bioflavonoids, zinc

Soft Tissue – A, B1, B2, C, niacin, pantothenic acid, calcium, zinc, silicon, manganese

Glands – A, pantothenic acid, choline, calcium, iodine

Enzymes – B6, magnesium, phosphorus, zinc, manganese, molybdenum

Growth – A, B1, B2, B12, biotin, folic acid, PABA, inositol, calcium, zinc, iodine

Metabolism – B1, B2, B6, B12, niacin, biotin, PABA, calcium, phosphorus, zinc, copper, manganese, iodine

Reproduction – A, B2, B12, E, zinc

Nerves – B1, B6, B12, niacin, pantothenic acid, choline, folic acid, PABA, calcium, magnesium, sodium, potassium, copper, manganese, cobalt, chlorine

Heart – B1, C, E, choline, folic acid, magnesium, potassium, selenium, chromium, silicon, cobalt

Blood – B2, B6, B12, E, niacin, folic acid, bioflavonoids, PABA, iron, copper, silicon, cobalt

Blood Clotting – C, E, K, folic acid, bioflavonoids, calcium, zinc, copper, manganese

Blood Pressure – choline, magnesium, sodium

Liver – B1, B2, E, choline, inositol, chromium, molybdenum

Brain – niacin, inositol, calcium, chlorine

Mental Processes – B1, B2, B6, B12, C, E, niacin, pantothenic acid, folic acid, copper

Memory – C, E, copper

Lungs – B6, calcium, magnesium

Kidneys – B6, C, calcium

RNA/DNA – B6, B12, biotin, folic acid, selenium

Immunity – A, B6, C, choline, folic acid, inositol, zinc, copper, iron, selenium, chromium, chlorine

Energy – B1, B2, E, pantothenic acid, copper, iron, chromium, cobalt, strontium

Menses, Menopause, PMS – B6, E, bioflavonoids

137

Vitamin/Mineral Help (con't.)

Pregnancy – A, B1, B2, B6, C, D, E, pantothenic acid, folic acid, bioflavonoids, calcium, magnesium, zinc, copper, iron, iodine, cobalt

Weight – B1, niacin

Aging – A, B1, B6, C, D, E, pantothenic acid, folic acid, calcium, phosphorus, zinc, chromium

Sleep – niacin, pantothenic acid, biotin

Toxins – A, C, E, pantothenic acid, choline, folic acid, sulfur, molybdenum

Smoking – A, C

Alcohol – B1, B2, B6, B12, C, D, niacin, pantothenic acid, biotin, choline, folic acid, phosphorus, potassium, zinc

Stress – A, B1, C, E, pantothenic acid

Radiation – Pantothenic acid

Allergies – E, pantothenic acid

Acne – B6, zinc

Cholesterol – C, niacin, inositol, zinc, chromium, silicon

Diabetes – B6, C, E, bioflavonoids, chromium

Cancer – A, B6, C, D, E, choline, PABA, inositol, selenium, chromium, silicon

Seizures – magnesium, chromium, manganese

Leg Cramps – B1, B6, E, pantothenic acid, calcium, sodium, potassium

Children – B12, C, folic acid, zinc, iron, cobalt, fluorine, protein

Athletes – B1, B2, niacin, iron, copper, selenium, protein

Vegetarian/Vegan – A, B6, B12, zinc, iron, cobalt, sulfur, protein

The Poor – B12, C, pantothenic acid, folic acid, phosphorus, potassium, zinc, protein

Addendum F
Coenzyme Q10

A new fat-soluble substance that acts like a vitamin is in the news lately. I wanted to give you what information was currently available and, like all nutrition information, more will be known as research continues. CoQ10 is present in most cells as part of the system of cellular respiration which generates 95% of the human body's energy.

A deficiency of coenzyme Q10, or CoQ10, seems to lead to premature aging. Statin drugs, like the kind used with regulating blood pressure and cholesterol, and chronic disease conditions can reduce the levels of CoQ10 by up to 40%. A deficiency is associated with heart disease, diabetes, periodontal disease, and stomach ulcers.

There seems to be no toxicity problem and up to 3600 mg has been tolerated by healthy adults. Any adverse effects in sensitive individuals have been related so far to gastrointestinal upsets (nausea, vomiting, stomachache). CoQ10 is best taken with food if used as a supplement, particularly foods that have a fat, since it is fat-soluble.

To date, CoQ10 is sold as a dietary supplement but is not approved by the FDA for the treatment of any medical condition. It is not regulated as a drug, but as a food. If you already take prescription medications, it is always wise to know what the interactions of vitamins and minerals will be with those. CoQ10 might interfere with the drug warfarin (Coumadin) because the structure of CoQ10 is similar to that of vitamin K, which competes with warfarin.

CoQ10 is also an antioxidant which supports the body's immune system by compromising free radicals, and in addition, seems to be an agent that regenerates other fat-soluble antioxidants, like vitamin E. Highest concentrations are in organs like the heart, liver, and kidneys, so it would have to benefit the health of those organs.

So far, these are the foods identified that contain CoQ10: beef, pork, chicken hearts, fish, coconut and olive oils, nuts, parsley, broccoli, cauliflower, spinach, grapes, Chinese cabbage, avocado, strawberries, oranges, grapefruit, apples, bananas. Meat and fish are the richest sources. Dairy, most fruits and berries except avocado are considered poor sources. An assumed daily intake is from 3-6 mg/day, mostly from meat.

There is some connection with niacin, with tryptophan, an essential amino acid in meat and fish, resveratrol in red wine, and one of the components found in blueberries. In combination, these three do most of the work. The trigger, however, the catalyst, is calorie reduction. You have to eat less.

The scientist who has done the latest research on this (vitamin?), a Harvard Medical School geneticist, David Sinclair, feels there is a potentially reversible cause of aging, and he became one of Time Magazine's 100 most influential men in the world because of his 2013 study. Sinclair is also supported in his claims by five Nobel prize winners. Because a deficiency has been linked to heart disease by another scientist who won a Nobel prize for that discovery, I have to believe that CoQ10 is also good for the heart. That would suggest a benefit for blood sugar regulation, tooth and gum health, and for stomach ulcers.

Glossary

Acid/alkaline referring to pH balance in the body, a number system between 0 – 14, 7 being the median, 7.4 being the average or normal for human bodies. Generally, lower than 6.9 is dangerous acidosis, and higher than 7.8 is dangerous alkalosis. (see chap. 6)

Acidosis/alkalosis refers to conditions leading to possible seizures, coma, and death.

Acne is an inflammatory disease of the sebaceous glands (near pores) and hair follicles of the skin that can scar the areas it affects.

Aerobic means living only in the presence of oxygen.

Allergies are due to an acquired hypersensitivity to a substance that normally would not produce a reaction.

Aluminum is a metal *and* a mineral. It is described in the mineral chapter (chap. 4). The human body needs a certain amount of aluminum in trace amounts, but with the way it is used in medicine, cookware, foil wrap, rain cloud seeding, and so forth, it is easy to get an overdose. The overdose seems to happen because of the way in which individual bodies absorb the mineral. Aluminum molecules attach to brain cells and are suspected in diseases like Alzheimers.

Alzheimers Disease is a form of dementia involving progressive, irreversible loss of memory and deterioration of intellectual functions.

AMA (American Medical Association) is the national organization which oversees health in all of its forms.

Amino acids are the building blocks of protein. Approximately 20 are required for human metabolism or growth, some supplied by food, the others produced by the body. Some proteins contain all of the essential amino acids and are called complete proteins. Among them are milk, cheese, eggs, and meat. Examples of incomplete proteins are vegetables and grains.

Anomalies are irregularity or deviations from the norm.

Antibiotics are any of a variety of natural or synthetic substances that inhibit growth of or destroy microorganisms used in the treatment of infectious diseases.

Antibodies belong to a group of serum proteins that respond to the threat of a foreign body and which form the basis for the body's immunity.

Antioxidant is an agent that prevents or inhibits destructive oxidation that can lead to disease states.

Apnea, Sleep is a temporary cessation of breathing, normally during sleep, which is the body's way of creating more CO_2 and an acidic state in the pursuit of pH balance. Consistent apnea can adversely complicate heart and kidney disease, brain injury, coma, and arteriosclerosis.

Arthritis is inflammation of a joint accompanied by pain and swelling, often disfigurement. It will also show up in other areas where bone has been injured.

Ascorbic acid is another name for Vitamin C.

Asthma is a sudden, periodic attack of labored or difficult breathing.

Astringent properties are agents that have a constricting or binding effect, such as in coagulation.

Atherosclerosis is a form of arteriosclerosis where fat and other substances accumulate in the arteries, posing a health risk.

Atrophy means to deteriorate or decay, a breaking down of a once healthy body part.

Autism is a condition resembling a self-centered mental state that characteristically includes an area of genius or high function. Those with autism, usually children, don't look you in the eye, are easily frightened by loud noise and aggressive behavior, they are severely introverted, and speak little. Fits are common and they never lie.

Autoimmune Disease is caused by something that compromises the immune system so that it can't respond, or responds inappropriately, to a threat to one's health. Generally, the body attacks itself. Examples of autoimmune diseases are Fibromyalgia, Chronic Fatigue Syndrome, Lupus, MS, and Rheumatoid Arthritis.

Beriberi is a disease caused by a deficiency of thiamine (see thiamine). Common during wartime with prisoners who ate only white rice.

Bilirubin is the orange-colored or yellowish pigment in bile, which is manufactured in the liver and stored in the gall bladder.

Biotin is a B complex vitamin, now called B7, formerly known as vitamin H. It plays a key role in the metabolism of fats, proteins, and carbohydrates.

Broad spectrum means that a particular vitamin or mineral will cover a lot of bases, will assist in many processes, a multi-tasker.

Bronchial dialation is a sympathetic nervous system response to labored breathing by sending a dilatory impulse to the bronchial muscles.

Bruxism is the gnashing or grinding of teeth, usually at night in one's sleep.

Buffers are part of the pH response to maintain acid/base balance, chiefly in the blood. (see ch. 6)

Cancer is a malignant tumor that can quickly spread to surrounding tissues by mutating cells.

Carcinogenic means it causes cancer.

Carotene is a yellow pigment found in various plant and animal tissues, and stored in the liver where it is converted to vitamin A.

Catalyst refers to something that begins a process, like when heat from the stove causes water to boil. Heat is the catalyst in that example. Another term for what it does might be called "jumpstarting."

Cataracts are opaque areas or spots of shadiness on the lens of the eye, on its capsule, or both.

Celiac Disease is an intestinal malabsorption problem characterized by bleeding tendency, diarrhea, malnutrition, and low calcium level. An intolerance to the gluten in grains.

Chlorophyll is the green pigment in plants that accompanies photosynthesis.

Chronic Fatigue Syndrome is one of the autoimmune diseases. It is a long-standing severe and disabling fatigue that has no cure.

Chronic Illness is long-term sickness, usually for life as there is no cure for most chronic conditions. That means a person who suffers with chronic illness does so every hour of every day, which is exhausting.

Cirrhosis is a chronic disease of the liver resulting in loss of functioning liver cells and increased resistance to flow of blood through the liver. The liver is one of the body's organs that will regenerate itself if the offending substance, i.e. drugs and alcohol, is discontinued.

Cleft palate occurs when the two bones of the upper jaw do not unite to form a continuous bone in fetal development resulting in an opening between the mouth and nasal cavities that can be repaired surgically.

Cobalamin is another name for vitamin B12.

Coenzyme is an enzyme activator and, when combined with an inactive protein, it forms a complete enzyme.

Collagen is the main supportive protein of skin, bone, tendon, cartilage, and connective tissue, representing about 30% of the body's protein.

Conjunctivitis is an inflammation of the mucous membranes that line the eyelids, one form of which is commonly called "pinkeye."

Corporate America is a term that refers to all large corporations that, in the case of food, determine the quality and quantity of our food supply and the laws that govern food production.

Cortisone an adrenal gland hormone which regulates metabolism of fats, carbohydrates, proteins, sodium, and potassium. It is also used as an anti-inflammatory agent.

Dementia is caused by organic brain disease and is characterized by irrecoverable deterioration of mental state and intellectual faculties.

Dermatitis is inflammation of the skin.

Detoxing is the process of ridding the body of toxic substances, that is, poisons. This is mainly done through exercise, nutrition, and fasting, once the toxic substances are discontinued.

Diabetes usually refers to diabetes mellitus recognized because of excessive urination. A disorder of carbohydrate metabolism resulting from inadequate production or utilization of insulin.

Diabetic Retinitis is inflammation of the retina in the eyes due to diabetes, especially long-term. Can lead to blindness.

Dilation means to increase in size or open up.

Diuretics are substances that ask your body to lose water, such as caffeine and water-soluble vitamins. If a person drinks coffee and/or takes supplements, for instance, it is then necessary to replace the water lost through urination.

Diuretic thiazide is often the first drug given to treat high blood pressure. Helps blood vessels to dilate, helps kidneys release salt and water, thus reducing fluid volume and lowering blood pressure.

DNA stands for deoxyribonucleic acid, a complex protein that is the chemical basis of heredity and the carrier of genetic information for all organisms.

Down's syndrome is a preferred term for mongolism, a variety of congenital moderate-to-severe mental retardation.

Electrolytes are solutions that are conductors of electricity. Acids, bases, and salts are common electrolytes in the human body.

Electromagnetic polarity refers to a positive (+), negative (-), or neutral effect of opposite poles, for instance, on a magnet or in a human cell. Electricity is able to travel based on the idea of polarity.

EMF's, or electromotive forces, are electrical flows from one place to another, to keep it simple, and can also refer to the energy field generated from such a flow.

Enzymes are complex proteins that are capable of inducing chemical changes in other substances without being changed themselves. They are present in digestive juices where they act upon food substances, causing them to break down into simpler compounds.

Epilepsy is a pattern of recurrent seizures, sudden brief attacks of altered consciousness, motor activity, or sensory phenomena, caused by many things like brain lesion, metabolic disturbances, toxic agents, or birth defect.

Estrogen Replacement Therapy refers to the taking of the female hormone, estrogen, orally to relieve the symptoms of menopause for women who have a uterus. It is considered a temporary treatment, as after 4 years of treatment there are decided risks. Taking this treatment should be carefully considered because of side effects and it will not be good for all women. It is an individual response that determines if it will work.

Excretion is the elimination of unused substances and water from the body. Toxins are carried out of the body by this process.

Fat-soluble refers to vitamins that are stored in the fat of the body to be used as needed.

FDA, or the Food & Drug Administration, is a regulatory body for foods, drugs, cosmetics, and medical devices. They regulate requirements for vitamins and minerals.

Fetus/Fetal has to do with a baby that is still in the womb, carried by its mother until birth takes place. This is a critical period for nutrition as deficiencies account for many birth defects. Alcohol, smoking, and drugs also contribute developmental abnormalities in the fetus.

Fibromyalgia is an autoimmune disease that has no cure involving chronic pain in the muscles and connective tissue that continually fluctuates between moderate and severe on a daily basis, and moves unpredictably around the body. No two victims will be found to have the same symptoms, but all can be diagnosed using the same characteristics.

Folic acid is also called folicin, B9, and folate. It is part of the B complex vitamins found naturally in green plant tissue, liver, and yeast. Used in the treatment of sprue, in the metabolism of nucleic acids and amino acids, for the production of red blood cells, and for normal cell division, especially during pregnancy and infancy which are times of rapid growth.

Food pyramids are a creation of the FDA and change periodically, so they are nothing more than a guide to nutritious eating, an attempt to balance food groups, etc. These guides follow a national philosophy of food consumption that is partially based on science and partially based on appeasing food lobbyists, such as the ones representing the wheat and dairy industries. They provide guides for us, but sometimes their guides lack common sense and individual needs and requirements. There is no substitute for doing your own thinking.

FTC stands for the federal trade commission and they regulate the advertising of food products, so they would be responsible for what is listed on food labels.

Gallstones are a mixture of cholesterol, bilirubin, and protein formed in the gall bladder or bile ducts. Painful when excreted through the ducts.

Gastrectomy is surgical removal of a part or the whole of the stomach.

Genetic disorder is a disorder of any part of the body if it is initiated by hereditary factors.

Glucose, or blood sugar, formed during digestion and is the most important carbohydrate in body metabolism. Level kept in check by insulin.

Gluten is a protein that can be prepared from wheat and other grain.

Gluten intolerance (see celiac disease) is an allergic reaction, possibly with a genetic component, to gluten, which is present in a large number of foods, especially where thickening sauces are used. Avoidance of gluten foods, such as wheat, rye, oats, and barley is essential.

GMO refers to genetically modified foods and foods grown from genetically modified seeds. GMO foods have been banned in 67 countries around the world, but for some reason (money), they are not illegal in the United States as of this writing. It is suspected that GMO's have the ability to alter DNA.

Goiter is an enlargement of the thyroid gland believed due to a deficiency of iodine.

Habitual abortion is three or more consecutive spontaneous abortions.

Hemochromatosis is a genetic disorder where too much iron is absorbed resulting in an accumulation of iron in the body, a condition that can have very serious side effects.

Hemoglobin is the iron-containing pigment of the red blood cells and its function is to carry oxygen from the lungs to the tissues.

Hemolysis is the destruction of red blood cells because of a trauma causing the liberation of hemoglobin, which diffuses into the fluid surrounding the cells. Excretion of fluids turns the urine red and could result in death.

Holocaust refers to the extermination of 6,000,000 Jews by the Nazis during World War II.

Hyperactivity is overactivity, distractibility, impulsiveness, inability to concentrate, and aggressiveness usually in children and adolescents. Medical information seeks to find something physically wrong to explain this condition, like heredity or mental disturbance, but it is also possible for hyperactivity to be an allergic reaction to toxins in our environment, they are so prolific.

Hypertension is a higher blood pressure than that judged to be normal.

Immune system is the body's protection system, especially from infectious agents, and includes responses from the skin, intestinal cells, white blood cells, and certain glands, including lymph.

Impotence is inability of the male to achieve or maintain erection.

Inflammation is the reaction of tissue to injury.

International units (IU) are a standard set for vitamins, some hormones, enzymes, and biologicals such as vaccines for ease in communicating across international borders.

Intravenous means within or into a vein, referring to medical practice of introducing fluids into the bloodstream of a patient.

Jaundice is a yellowing of skin and tissues due to malfunctions of the liver and bile ducts which spill excess bilirubin into the blood.

Kidney stones are small to medium granular masses in the kidneys that are painful when excreted through the urinary canal.

Lactation is the function of secreting milk in the breasts of mammals, and including the period of suckling.

Lactic acid is a colorless liquid formed in milk and fermented foods, and also by the breakdown of glycogen during muscular activity.

Lactose intolerance is an intolerance to milk causing gastrointestinal symptoms. Pasteurization kills the lactose digestive enzyme which leads to an allergic reaction to milk because it can't be properly digested.

Legumes are, in the average experience, usually peas, beans, and peanuts.

Lesions an injury or a wound, or a single patch of infected skin.

Lupus is an autoimmune disease with ulcerating skin lesions on the face, neck, and upper extremities of unknown origin, sometimes accompanied by joint pain and malaise.

Lymph is a colorless, alkaline fluid, found in the lymphatic vessels, that carries bacteria and toxins away from where they could do harm.

Membranes are thin, soft layers of tissue that line a tube or cavity, that cover an organ or structure, or separate one part from another.

Menses, or menstruation, or period, the fairly regular discharge of the blood and mucous lining from the uterus from puberty to menopause in the life of a woman.

Metabolism is the sum of all physical and chemical changes that take place within an organism, all energy and material transformations that occur within living cells. The burning of fuel.

Metabolic disturbance can be diabetes mellitus or any other disorder related to metabolism.

Miscarriage is a lay term referring to the involuntary termination of any pregnancy after the fourth month.

Mitigation means moderated or diminished in severity.

Mongolism is another name for Down's syndrome or severe retardation.

Multiple sclerosis (MS) is an autoimmune disease with no cure and no known cause. A chronic, slowly progressive disease of the central nervous system.

Muscular dystrophy is a generalized wasting away, an atrophy and weakness of muscles.

Myelin sheath is composed of lipids (fats) and protein and forms a sheath or covering around the axons of certain nerves.

Myesthenia gravis is faulty nerve conduction resulting in a muscular weakness or fatigue, especially around the face and neck.

Neurotransmitters help to carry a nerve impulse across the synapse of a nerve cell.

Niacin, or nicotinic acid, is another name for vitamin B3.

Nitrates are salts of nitric acid, caustic, corrosive, poisonous.

Nitrites are salts of nitrous acid, have some medical uses.

Obesity is a condition characterized by excess body fat, often defined as 20% above desirable body weight. Just a guide. Keep in mind that extra weight is naturally put on in colder climates to protect the body, some people are big-boned and carry more weight, exercise builds muscle which weighs more, and some body types lend themselves to extra weight as long as mobility is not impaired and the lifestyle includes nutrition and exercise. The clue is that the weight causes your body to become sedentary, or it creates on-going health concerns. It is far more important to have peace of mind than to continually fear that you're not as good as others.

Omega 3's, linoleic acids, are fatty acids that the body cannot make so they must be ingested. They must be present in the diet to maintain good health. Omega 3's participate in immune function, and vision, help form cell membranes, and aid in the production of hormone-like compounds. They tend to decrease blood clotting and inflammatory responses.

Oral contraceptives or birth control pills.

Organic refers to carbon liked to hydrogen in the chemical structure. Organic food is chemical free, like farmer's market-type vegetables. Organic meat would mean no vaccines, hormones, processed feeds or other chemicals, grass fed or range free.

Osteoarthritis is a chronic disease involving the joints, especially weight-bearing joints, degenerative destruction of cartilage with impaired function.

Osteoporosis is softening and loss of bone seen most often in the elderly.

Oxalic acid is a naturally-occurring toxin in foods, found in spinach, cranberries, chard, rhubarb, gooseberries, beet leaves. It is a toxin because it binds calcium and prevents its uptake. All food groups have calcium, however, so just eat more calcium foods, such as eggs, beans, and milk, at a different time.

Oxidation is the process of a substance combining with oxygen. Utilization of oxygen by cells. The body is burning fuel.

Palpitations are rapid, throbbing, or fluttering pulsations, usually of the heart.

Pantothenic acid is another name for vitamin B5 which is used in the oxidation of fatty acids and carbohydrates, and also in the synthesis of amino acids, neurotransmitters, and antibodies, among others.

Pathological means a condition produced by disease.

Periodontal Disease is any abnormality of the tissue around the tooth.

Peristalsis is an involuntary wavelike movement, a simultaneous contraction and relaxation in the hollow tubes of the body, especially the alimentary canal where this method is used to move food along until the waste is excreted.

Permeability means the capability of allowing the passage of fluids or substances in solution; the penetration of a membrane or cell wall.

Pernicious anemia is a severe form of blood disease marked by a progressive decrease in red blood corpuscles, muscular weakness, and gastrointestinal and neural disturbances.

pH balance is a maintainence of the acidity and alkalinity of the fluids and electrolytes of the body. (see chap. 6)

Phlebitis is inflammation, pain, and tenderness along the course of a vein.

PMS, or premenstrual syndrome, occurs several days prior to the onset of menstruation, related to alterations in estrogen, which causes irritability, anxiety, emotional tension, mood swings, depression, among others.

Postpartum is that period occurring after childbirth.

Precursor is a substance that precedes another substance.

Predisposition is the potential to develop a certain disease or condition in the presence of specific environmental stimuli.

Premature infants are those who are born before the end of their full gestation time. Early birth.

Probiotics means good for, supportive of, or caused by life or living things.

Psoriasis is a common, itching dermatitis with lesions on the skin.

Pyridoxine is another name for vitamin B6. It is a coenzyme in many enzymatic reactions in metabolism.

Rancid means that partial decomposition has produced an offensive odor or taste.

Retardation is a delayed mental or physical response due to pathological conditions. A birth defect.

Rhetoric is language that is showy and elaborate but largely empty of clear ideas or sincere emotion.

Rheumatic heart disease is an acute or chronic inflammatory disease characterized by pain, fever, swelling of the joints, and inflammation of the heart.

Rheumatoid arthritis is an autoimmune disease of unknown cause or cure with pain, swelling, and inflammation of the joints leading to deformity of the joints.

Rheumatism is any of various painful conditions involving the joints and muscles with inflammation and stiffness.

Riboflavin is another name for vitamin B2. Helps activate other vitamins.

Rickets is a disease of the skeletal system where a softening and bending of the bones is the result of a deficiency of vitamin D, usually found in children. It resembles a bow-legged appearance from the knees down.

RNA, or ribonucleic acid, is a nucleic acid that is an essential component of all cells, controlling protein synthesis.

Salmonella is a bacteria-caused food poisoning.

Schizophrenia is a mental disorder with psychotic features representing a deterioration from a previous level of function, with delusions, hallucinations, or thought disturbances.

Scientific compartmentalization has to do with the way scientists act territorial in their specialty leading to a study of parts unrelated to the whole.

Sedentary lifestyle is one with minimal physical activity usually accompanied by weight gain.

Seizures are sudden attacks of pain, of a disease, or of certain symptoms, with abnormal brain wave patterns and brief loss of consciousness.

Sleep apnea is a periodic cessation of breathing during sleep.

Special circumstances are times when a diet needs to be modified because of things like pregnancy, childhood, aging, athleticism, or disease states.

Special interest manipulation is when those in the food industry, for example, try to pass laws or influence regulation of their products to increase profits. A recent example is the lobbying of congress to water down the word "organic" so that it can mean 70% organic. They wanted to use the word in advertising but knew their products would never be 100% chemical free. The law passed.

Spontaneous abortion means that a fetus was aborted from the uterus without apparent cause.

Sprue is a condition where there is a faulty absorption of fats and vitamins, esp. vitamin E. It manifests weakness and loss of weight, along with various digestive disorders.

Stillbirth is the birth of a dead fetus.

Sulpha drugs are drugs of the sulfonamide group possessing bacteriostatic properties, inhibiting or retarding the growth of bacteria.

Supplements are the pill form of vitamins and minerals used to bolster the nutritional content of the diet, for instance, when a vegan takes a cobalt supplement because cobalt is only found in animal sources in food.

Synthesis is the opposite of decomposition where more complex substances are formed from simpler elements; a building up.

Thiamine is another name for vitamin B1. It is essential for the normal metabolism of carbohydrates and fats.

Thiazide diuretics increase the amount of sodium and water that is re-absorbed by the kidneys.

Thrombosis is the formation, development, or existence of a blood clot within the vascular (blood vessels) system.

Tinnitus is what we call ringing in the ears.

Toxemia is poisonous products of bacteria growing in a local area and spreading throughout the body.

Toxins are poisonous substances of animal or plant origin, stored in the fat of the body.

Tuberculosis (TB) is an infectious disease affecting the respiratory system; can lead to death.

Varicose veins are enlarged and twisted veins close to the skin's surface accompanied by pain and swelling, possibly bruising, seen mostly in the lower extremities and esophagus.

Vegan is a person who eats food only from plant sources.

Vegetarian is a person who doesn't eat meat, but may eat things like eggs, milk, and yogurt.

Vertigo is a middle ear imbalance which causes one to feel like they are moving around in space. It is difficult to stand or walk and there is often nausea.

Water-soluble refers to vitamins that dissolve in water and are regularly passed out of the body and need to be replaced.

Wilson's disease is an increase of intestinal absorption of copper resulting in degenerative changes in the brain, cirrhosis of the liver, tremor, spastic contractures, muscle rigidity, psychic disturbances, and progressive weakness and emaciation.

Index

Blood clotting (wound healing, vit. K) 36, 38, 41, 44, 47, 53, 59, 60, 65
Blood pressure 35, 44, 55
Bones 21, 38, 43, 53, 54, 55, 56, 59, 64, 65, 68, 72
Brain 9, 28, 37, 38, 42, 53, 65, 67, 69, 75, 101
Bruxism 32, 33

C＿＿＿＿＿

Calcium 31, 33, 43, 52, 53-54, 55, 56, 61, 64, 72, 102
Cancer 3, 6, 21, 30, 35, 38, 40, 42, 43, 44, 62, 63, 64, 81, 105, 106, 109
Cataracts 26
Celiac disease 1, 89
Children 1, 37, 59, 61, 67, 68, 91, 108
Chlorine 52, 69
Cholesterol 29, 38, 42, 59, 63, 64, 97, 106, 115
Choline (vit. B4) 35
Chromium 52, 63
Chronic fatigue syndrome 37, 109
Cirrhosis 42, 45
Cleft palate 23
Cobalt 52, 67, 90
Colon 64, 82
Comfort foods 4, 83
Conjunctivitis 26
Copper 52, 59, 60, 71
Core food group 12
Core lifestyle 12, 110
Cramps, leg 24, 45
Cramps, menstrual 31
Cramps, muscle 53, 54, 57, 58

G_____

Gallstones 38, 107
Glands 21, 22, 32, 35, 53, 66
Glucose 34, 63
Gluten intolerance 11, 89, 110
GMO 80, 98, 109, 110
Goiter 66
Growth 21, 22, 24, 26, 28, 34, 36, 37, 40, 42, 59,
60, 66, 67, 101

H_____

Habitual abortion 44
Heart 23, 24, 31, 35, 36, 38, 44, 46, 55, 57, 58,
        62, 63, 64, 67, 82, 86, 105, 109, 118
Hormones 30, 66
Hyperactivity 12, 78, 91, 109
Hypertension 44, 55, 57, 69, 78, 79, 89, 102, 115

I_____

Immune system 20, 30, 35, 36, 38, 42, 59, 60, 61,
        69, 75, 106, 109, 117
Infection 21, 22, 32, 35, 36, 37, 38, 39, 59, 117
Inflammation 26, 34, 36, 54, 59, 105, 107
Inositol (vit. B8) 42, 90
Iodine 33, 66, 90, 102
Iron 30, 38, 59, 61, 71, 102

J_____

Junk food 76, 83, 84

K_____

Kidneys 55, 85-86, 87, 105, 107
Kidney stones 19, 30, 53

L

M

N

O

Osteoarthritis 32
Osteoporosis 53, 115

P_____

PABA (vit. B10) 40, 90
Palpitations (irregular heartbeat) 35, 36, 55, 58,
    67
Pancreas 45, 63
Pantothenic acid (vit. B5) 32-33, 102
Paralysis 24, 26, 35, 37
Pellagra 28
Periodontal disease 44, 53
Pernicious anemia 37, 67
Pesticides, herbicides, fungiscides, insecticides
    introduction, 8, 33, 108
Pets 27
pH balance 57, 58, 69, 70, 85-88
Phlebitis 45
Phosphorus 52, 56, 85
PMS (prémenstruel syndrome) 30
Postpartum 41
Potassium 30, 31, 52, 58, 105
Pregnancy 1, 13, 20, 21, 25, 31, 36, 37, 39, 44,
    51, 61, 66, 91, 101-103
Premature baby 36, 44, 56, 60
Psoriasis 42

R_____

Radiation 32, 72, 109
Reproductive health 21, 23, 26, 37, 44, 59
Research 7, 8, 13, 14-15, 39, 51, 84, 91
Retardation 32, 43, 66
Rheumatic heart disease 44
Rheumatoid arthritis 30, 32, 109
Rheumatism 30, 43
Riboflavin (vit. B2) 26-27, 102
Rickets 43, 53, 68
RNA (ribonucleic acid) 30, 37

S_____

Salmonella 34
Schizophrenia 29, 36
Sedentary lifestyle 19, 75, 86, 97
Seizures (convulsions) 30, 55, 63, 65, 108
Selenium 44, 45, 46, 62, 64
Silicon 52, 64, 90
Skin 21, 28, 30, 34, 40, 41, 44, 59, 90
Sleep disturbances 28, 32, 34, 53-54, 109
Smoking 3, 21, 39, 80, 82, 86
Sodium 52, 55, 57, 58, 69, 73, 79, 89
Soft tissue (membranes, connective tissue) 20, 21,
        22, 24, 28, 32, 38, 41, 44, 53, 56, 59, 64,
        65, 102
Spontaneous abortion 23, 41
Sprue 45
Stillbirth 32
Stress 5, 21, 25, 32, 45, 101, 109
Stroke 36, 57, 110
Strontium 52, 72
Sugar 9, 12, 25, 35, 54, 73, 78-79, 85, 90, 91, 96,
        98, 103, 108
Sulfur 52, 70, 85, 90
Sulpha drugs 34, 36, 40
Supplements, vitamin & mineral 19, 31, 45, 46,
        60, 65, 67, 90, 93, 101, 102, 106

T_____

Teeth 6, 21, 30, 38, 41, 53, 54, 56, 68, 71, 72,
        110
Thiamin (vit. B1) 24-25, 102
Thiazide diuretic 55
Thrombosis 41
Tinnitus 108
Toxemia 36
Toxins (pollution, poisons) 8, 12, 15, 21, 22, 32,
        35, 36, 38, 39, 43, 44, 51, 52, 63, 70, 81,
        97, 105, 106, 107, 108, 109, 110
TB (tuberculosis) 21, 109

V

Varicose veins 41, 44
Vegetarian/vegan 7, 8, 11, 22, 27, 37, 42, 56, 59, 61, 67, 70, 90, 91, 93, 97, 103
Vertigo 108
Vitamins 10, 11, 13, 19-47, 70, 80, 91, 102, 113-114
Vitamin A 19, 20, 21-22, 33, 44, 46
Vitamin B6 30-31, 55, 102
Vitamin B12 35, 37, 80, 90, 102
Vitamin C 10, 19, 20, 33, 38-39, 41, 46, 61, 78, 80
Vitamin D 19, 20, 43, 56, 90
Vitamin E 19, 20, 33, 44-46
Vitamin K 19, 20, 47, 65

W

Water 19, 22, 40, 78-79, 81-82, 93, 97, 102
Wilson's disease 60

Z

Zinc 52, 59, 61

www.ingramcontent.com/pod-product-compliance
Lightning Source LLC
Chambersburg PA
CBHW070840310526
45793CB00010B/119